EPIDEMIOLOGY

BASIS FOR DISEASE PREVENTION
AND HEALTH PROMOTION

David F. Duncan, Dr.P.H.

SOUTHERN ILLINOIS UNIVERSITY AT CARBONDALE

with the assistance of

Robert S. Gold, Ph.D., Dr.P.H.

U.S. OFFICE OF DISEASE PREVENTION AND HEALTH PROMOTION

Charles E. Basch, Ph.D.

TEACHER'S COLLEGE—COLUMBIA UNIVERSITY

Victoria C. Markellis, M.D., M.P.H.

STATE UNIVERSITY OF NEW YORK AT BROCKPORT

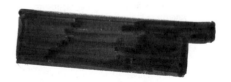

MACMILLAN PUBLISHING COMPANY

NEW YORK

Collier Macmillan Publishers

LONDON

This book is gratefully dedicated to

Reuel A. Stallones
for introducing me to the fascination and excitement
of epidemiology as only a great teacher could.

Blair Justice and Cornelius Askew
for encouraging me to explore the breadth of
epidemiology and to push against its accepted
boundaries.

Bill Zimmerli, John Sinacore, and Don Boydston
for their consistent support and encouragement of my
teaching and research in epidemiology.

Macmillan Publishing Company
866 Third Avenue, New York, New York 10022

Collier Macmillan Canada, Inc.

LIBRARY OF CONGRESS CATALOGING-IN-PUBLICATION DATA
Duncan, David F.
   Epidemiology: basis for disease prevention and
health promotion.
   Bibliography: p.
   Includes index.
   1. Epidemiology—Popular works. I. Title.
[DNLM: 1. Epidemiology—popular works. WA 105 D911e]
RA653.D86 1987   614.4   86-23854
ISBN 0-02-330840-0

Printing: 1 2 3 4 5 6 7   Year: 8 9 0 1 2 3 4

ISBN   0-02-330840-0

About the Author

David Duncan received the degree of Doctor of Public Health (Dr.P.H.) from the University of Texas School of Public Health in Houston, Texas. His doctoral training emphasized the areas of epidemiology, biostatistics, and mental health. His major professor was Dr. Blair Justice, and his mentor in epidemiology was Dr. Reuel Stallones. He received his introduction to psychiatric epidemiology from Dr. Cornelius Askew.

His undergraduate education included an Associate in Science degree from the Metropolitan Junior College of Kansas City, with a double major in biology and social science, and a Bachelor of Arts degree from the University of Missouri at Kansas City, with a major in psychology. He subsequently attended Sam Houston State University in Huntsville, Texas, where he completed 36 hours of graduate course work in criminology. He also earned certification in counseling and therapy for alcoholism, drug abuse, and related disorders at the University of Houston.

He is currently Professor of Health Education and Coordinator of the Community Health Program at Southern Illinois University at Carbondale. Prior to this position, he was Associate Professor of Health Science at the State University of New York College at Brockport. During Fall of 1986 he spent a sabbatical as Visiting Professor of Health and Environmental Research at the University of Cologne in Cologne, West Germany. He is a member of the Society for Epidemiologic Research, the American College of Epidemiology, the Society for Clinical Trials and the American Public Health Association. He is a past-Chairman of the Mental Health Section of the American Public Health Association.

As a scholar and researcher he is the author or coauthor of over forty papers published in scientific journals and of two books. Most of his epidemiologic research has focused on two areas: drug abuse and family violence. He has also conducted research on other epidemiologic topics such as rheumatoid arthritis, chronic obstructive airway disorders, heart disease, suicide, and the mental health of the elderly.

Preface

Despite its serious and often unpleasant subject matter, epidemiology is for me the most exciting of the sciences. It shares with all the sciences the rigorous pleasures of observation, the rewarding effort of analysis, and the joy of discovery. But it does so with subject material that is among the closest to the everyday life of humanity. The potential for improving the quality of human lives may be greater for epidemiology than for any other science.

In the chapters ahead, the student will learn about the historical and theoretical bases of epidemiology; the statistical methods used in epidemiology; the distribution of disease over person, place, and time; the research methods used in analytic epidemiology; and the application of epidemiology to the prevention of disease and the promotion of health.

I can only hope that the text will convey to the student some of the excitement that the field holds for me. Epidemiology is not a dull subject. It is a lively one because it is vitally concerned with human life.

D. F. D.

Contents

Prolog

The Epidemiologic Approach
and the Uses of Epidemiology

In 1976, public attention was focused on Philadelphia not only because of the bicentennial of the signing of the Declaration of Independence but also because of a mysterious epidemic of pneumonia that struck there soon after the Fourth of July. An apparently new disease[1] had struck 221 people at Philadelphia's Bellevue-Stratford Hotel, many of whom were attending an American Legion Convention—thus giving rise to the name "Legionnaires' Disease," or Legionellosis, for this virulent pneumonia. A majority of the cases occurred within a 12-day interval, and 6.8 percent of the conventioneers developed the disease. Thirty-four persons (16 percent of the cases) died.

It was through the news coverage of this investigation that many Americans first heard of that small band of scientists known as *epidemiologists*. Although the expected white lab coats and microscopes were very much in evidence among some of the scientists searching out the causes of this epidemic, the epidemiologists did not conduct their investigation in the fashion most people expected. Instead of working with test tubes and microscopes in laboratories, they spent their time asking people questions and poking into every corner of the hotel—

---

[1] It was eventually learned that previously there had been at least two smaller epidemics of the same disease—one in Washington, D.C. in 1965 and the other at the same Philadelphia hotel in 1974. There had also been previous epidemics of Pontiac Fever, a nonpneumonic disease caused by the same bacteria as Legionnaires' Disease.

even examining the contents of the waste baskets. Stranger still, they seemed as interested in the people who did not get sick as in those who did—even surveying American Legion members who had decided not to attend the convention. It is the comparison of groups (e.g., the sick with the well, attenders with nonattenders) that is the essence of the epidemiologic approach.

When a group of people gathered for an occasion such as a convention are stricken by an epidemic illness, food poisoning is always suspected. Epidemiologists soon found, however, that there was no association between eating at certain convention functions or at certain restaurants and occurrence of the disease. The possibility of contaminated water supply is also a consideration and the investigators did find a statistically significant association between consumption of drinking water at the hotel and occurrence of the disease. However, of 69 ill delegates from whom information was obtained, 24 had not consumed any water at the Bellevue-Stratford Hotel. Epidemiologists concluded that the association simply represented the fact that those who had spent more time at the hotel were more likely to have consumed some water there, while it was the amount of time spent in the hotel that was causally linked with the disease.

The possibility of person-to-person transmission of the disease was also examined by the epidemiologists. They found that persons who had shared a room with someone who developed the disease were not significantly more likely to develop the disease than those with a disease-free roommate. Likewise, there was no evidence of transmission of the disease to family members by cases who had returned home before becoming ill.

The possibility that the disease was airborne was suggested to the epidemiologists by the higher frequency of the disease among Legionnaires staying at the Bellevue-Stratford than among those staying elsewhere in Philadelphia. This was more strongly indicated when surveys of both ill and well Legionnaires revealed that among Legionnaires who did not stay at the Bellevue-Stratford, the frequency of the disease was higher among those who had spent more time in the lobby of the hotel. Cases even occurred in persons who had not entered the hotel but who had spent time on the sidewalk in front of the hotel where air from the lobby passed out through the front door.

Acting on the basis of this evidence, epidemiologists isolated the disease organism now known as *Legionella pneumophila* in water from the hotel's air-conditioning system cooling tower. The organism showed a striking ability to survive in sterile water and was likely to thrive in conditions of elevated temperature and in which organic matter is present in a cooling tower. As air passes through a cooling tower in the heat-exchange process, a cloud of droplets (known as "drift") is generated, which can be expected to contain any bacteria present in the cooling tower water. This "drift" may be disseminated over a wide area and in some cases may be drawn into the air-conditioning system itself through its air intakes, thus spreading *L. pneumophila* throughout the air-conditioned area.

The Epidemiologic Approach ───────────────────────

Like the names of most sciences, the term *epidemiology* is derived from Greek root words. *Epi* for upon—as in epidermis, the layer of dead skin cells on top of the dermis, the living skin. *Demos* for the people—as in democracy. *Logos* for thought or study—as in logic or biology. Thus, epidemiology is the study of that which befalls the people; the study of the diseases, accidents, and disasters that befall us all.

The epidemiologic approach to the study of these events is rooted in the basic assumption that these events do not befall the population in a purely random or chance fashion. When two populations differ in the extent to which they suffer from a disease, an epidemiologist presumes that some other difference between the communities is causally related to the disease. In short, epidemiologists believe in causes—not in luck—as the determiner of who gets sick.

Keeping this assumption in mind we can begin to define epidemiology more precisely. Lilienfeld (1978) found that epidemiology is defined in a variety of different ways by different authors. The one commonality seems to be the frequent use of the phrase, "the distribution of." By the distribution of disease, for instance, we mean that an epidemiologist wants to know what groups of people, places, and time suffer greatly from a disease, and what characteristics high-rate groups may have in common. Consistent with Lilienfeld's review, we propose the following definition: Epidemiology is the study of the distribution and determinants of the varying rates of diseases, injuries, or other health states in human populations.

David Lilienfeld (1978) proposed a new definition of epidemiology: "Epidemiology is a method of reasoning about disease that deals with biological inferences derived from observations of disease phenomena in population groups" (p. 89). Lilienfeld's definition has much to recommend it, but it also incorporates two assumptions about the scope of epidemiology that this author finds objectionable: that epidemiology is only concerned with (1) disease and (2) biological inferences about disease. Although both statements might have been accurate about epidemiology as it was practiced a half-century ago, the scope of contemporary epidemiology has been expanded to include injuries and other nondisease health states, and is increasingly coming to encompass psychological and sociological inferences in its examination of its subject matter.

In examining the burden of disease on any community, an epidemiologist is always concerned with rates of disease—with the proportion of the population that is affected by the disease. In subsequent chapters we will examine a variety of rates that are used by epidemiologists. At this point we will discuss two rates that are widely used in epidemiology: the *incidence rate* and the *prevalence rate*.

Incidence is a measure of the rate at which new events occur in a population. The numerator of this rate is the number of new events (usually the number of newly diagnosed or reported cases of a particular disease) occurring during a specified period of time. The denominator is the "population at risk," the total number of persons in the community who could have experienced the new event (who could have become new cases of the disease). Ideally, then, this is a population figure that excludes persons who already have the disease or who could not possibly have developed the disease. In actual practice, however, the total population is usually used as the population-at-risk denominator because the number of persons within the population who are not at risk is usually unknown. The result of this division is multiplied by a constant (some power of 10, such as 1,000 or 100,000) to obtain a whole number:

$$\text{Incidence} = \frac{\text{Number of new events during time period}}{\text{Population at risk}} \times 1,000$$

Prevalence is a measure of the proportion of the population experiencing an event (usually a disease) at a designated time or during a given time period—in the former case it is known as *point prevalence;* in the latter case it is known as *period prevalence*. The prevalence rate takes this form:

$$\text{Prevalence} = \frac{\text{Number of events (both new and old)}}{\text{Population at risk}} \times 1,000$$

Uses of Epidemiology ————————————————————————

What is the value of such an examination of diseases, injuries, or health states? J. N. Morris (1975) has identified seven uses of epidemiology that provide the basis for the discussion that follows. These uses are not necessarily unique to epidemiology; some of them are shared with other biomedical sciences. The special importance of epidemiology in this regard is that it places the findings of other disciplines into perspective, considering disease as a population-based phenomenon in an environmental context.

First and foremost, epidemiology is concerned with identifying the causes of disease, as in the case of Legionnaires' Disease recounted earlier. Epidemiology shares this function to some degree with the fields of pathology, microbiology, biochemistry, and the other biomedical sciences, but epidemiology differs in the breadth of its approach and in the use of population-based methods. This has allowed epidemiology to develop more complex models with which to explain disease causation in a manner that better fits the real world than do laboratory-based models. Epidemiologic methods have also been applied to the study of causation of nondisease entities, such as traffic accidents or murders.

Second, epidemiology completes the clinical picture of a disease. This refers to the fact that physicians (or others who treat disease) inevitably have a distorted view of the nature and distribution of the disease. This is in part because persons with mild cases of a disease are less likely to seek treatment, thus making clinicians likely to overestimate the severity of the disease. An example is found in the medical literature on the abuse of the drug PCP, or phencyclidine. It is difficult to understand why anyone would want to take a drug that can cause paranoia, violent and sometimes self-destructive behavior, respiratory difficulties, coma, and, in some cases, death. The point is, however, that these effects of PCP are relatively rare, but they are the effects that bring PCP users to emergency rooms where they are observed by physicians, and thus they have formed the clinical picture of PCP abuse.

In part, the distortions of the clinical picture arise from the fact that we are not all equally likely to seek medical care when we are ill. Women, for instance, are more likely than men to seek medical care for the same condition. This can lead physicians to falsely conclude that certain conditions are more common among women simply because they see more women with the disease. Similarly, the poor generally must be sicker before they will seek medical care than the rich. This may cause physicians to falsely conclude that some diseases are less common among the poor than among the rich. Alternately, it could cause physicians to falsely assume that the disease is, in fact, a more severe disease when it occurs among the poor. Distortions may also result from differences in access to diagnosis and treatment. An interesting example is provided by the early reports on child abuse, which identified this problem as being almost entirely associated with poverty. In fact, we now know that child abuse is almost as common in wealthy families as in poor families. When we first became concerned with child abuse, however, most cases were being identified through routine x-ray procedures in hospital emergency rooms. Parents of lower-class status who had injured their children were more likely to take them to the emergency room for treatment where the abuse would be identified. Parents of upper-class status were more likely to take their child to a family physician, who was likely to identify abuse as the cause of the child's injuries or to report the abuse even if it was apparent.

Third, epidemiology has allowed us to identify syndromes—to "lump and split" related conditions into groups that make scientific and clinical sense. For instance, the traditional division of diabetes mellitus into categories of juvenile-onset diabetes and adult-onset diabetes has been replaced by the similar but more clinically useful distinction between insulin-dependent and insulin-independent diabetes. Similarly, epidemiologists have been able to identify varieties of hepatitis and behavioral groupings of juvenile delinquents that have great relevance both for enhancing our understanding of causation and for developing effective treatment methods.

Fourth, epidemiologic methods can be applied to determining the effectiveness of therapeutic and preventive measures. The procedures by which new drugs must be tested for safety and effectiveness before they can be marketed in the U.S. are essentially epidemiologic procedures. Unfortunately, many common medical procedures have never been tested in any truly scientific manner to determine their effectiveness. In recent years, however, epidemiologic methods have been used to set a standard for the groups of women who should have periodic mammography (breast x-rays) for the detection of breast cancer—weighing the value for each group of early detection against the risk that the x-rays may cause the cancer. Epidemiologic studies have cast serious doubt on the value of coronary bypass surgery for many, perhaps most, patients undergoing this increasingly common surgery.

Fifth, epidemiology provides the means with which to monitor the health of a community, region, or nation. It can identify the health problems of greatest importance and the target populations most appropriate for intervention. Rational health planning is made possible by an epidemiologic data base.

Sixth, risks identified for groups by epidemiologists can be applied to the individual members of those groups as probability statements. This is the basis for the health hazard appraisals that have become so popular in recent years. Although many doubts exist about the validity of such predictions for individuals rather than groups, and about the value of such predictions as ways to motivate behavior, this use has achieved great popularity among health educators and program planners concerned with changing health behavior.

Seventh, by studying trends over time in the history of a disease, it is possible to make predictions about the future. The relative stability of accidental death rates over more than three-quarters of a century suggests that neither lowered speed limits nor elevated drinking ages will have much effect on death rates because the raising of speed limits and the lowering of drinking ages had no apparent effect in the past. On the other hand, reducing federal funding for immunization programs predictably is followed by measles epidemics that leave a few children unnecessarily blind, deaf, brain damaged, or dead.

Historical studies may also contribute to our understanding of the causes of disease. An outstanding example of a historical pattern that suggests a causal relationship is the increase in lung cancer mortality in relation to increasing cigarette smoking. Another historical application of epidemiology that has grown in recent years is the study of the influence of disease patterns on social and political history. Was the plague the primary cause of the fall of the Roman Empire (by decimating the Roman army and disrupting the Roman economy)? Was Napoleon defeated more by typhus among his troops and by his own hemmorhoids than by the military forces allied against him? Historians such as Zinsser (1942) and Cartwright (1972) have speculated that disease patterns may in fact have influenced greatly social and political history.

As can be seen by the brief overview given, epidemiology has many uses. As epidemiologic methods have been applied to an ever broadening array of problems, the range of potential uses has grown. This growth may only be at its beginning stages today.

Recommended Reading

Morris, J. N. (August 13, 1955). Uses of epidemiology. *British Medical Journal*, 2, 395–401.

Morris, J. N. (1975). *Uses of epidemiology* (3rd ed.). New York: Churchill Livingstone.

Public Health Reports. (1980). *Landmarks in American epidemiology, 95*(2). Special issue.

Stallones, R. A. (1980). To advance epidemiology. *Annual Review of Public Health, 1,* 69–82.

PART I

Background to Epidemiology

To those who say, "How can we admit the possibility of infection while the religious law denies it," we reply that the existence of contagion is established by experience, investigation, the evidence of the senses and trustworthy reports. These facts constitute a sound argument. The fact of infection becomes clear to the investigator who notices how he who establishes contact with the afflicted gets the disease, whereas he who is not in contact remains safe, and how transmission is effected through garments, vessels and earrings.

— *Ibn-al-Khatib, 14th-century Moorish scholar*

To understand any contemporary science it is necessary to have some understanding of its roots. Chapter 1 provides a historical overview of changing concepts of the causation of disease. Epidemiologic methods originally developed in an attempt to compensate for the failures of germ theory in the explanation of infectious disease. Gradually, epidemiologic theory grew from the infectious disease oriented model of classic epidemiologic theory (Chapter 2). Today, epidemiology provides a theoretical framework for health service, including disease prevention and health promotion.

CHAPTER 1

Mankind's Changing Concepts of Disease

It is the purpose of this chapter to provide the reader with an introduction to the variety of ways in which our ancestors attempted to explain the causes of disease. A historical perspective such as this can provide a valuable insight into many current beliefs about health and disease. It is hoped that such a perspective will also inspire some humility regarding our own certainties as we examine the false conceptions that have been accepted in the past.

Such a brief history of the concepts of disease necessarily omits a great deal. The reader should be aware that theories of disease causation were not replaced by others in a neat and orderly progression. Instead, they frequently overlapped and coexisted. Today, we still view the elements of these theories in popular ideas about disease and in the practice of medicine.

Primitive Peoples' Concepts of Disease

Early man attributed disease to the actions of evil spirits or ghosts. Alternately, it was believed that disease could be the result of witchcraft—a curse or an "evil eye" put on the disease victim by an enemy. Disease, like famine, drought, or lightning, was believed to be an act of the supernatural, beyond human control or human understanding.

To prevent disease, one made sacrifices to the gods, obeyed the taboos, and avoided haunted places. Charms and spells were also used to protect one from disease. These primitive notions still exist to some extent today. In the midst of our modern cities, one can still find those who by charms, amulets, and potions will guarantee to prevent or cure disease, to bring you your true love, or to give you luck at gambling.

The Hippocratic–Galenic Theory

The First Epidemiologist

The Greek Physician Hippocrates of Cos, who lived from about 460 B.C. until about 377 B.C., was the earliest known authority to attempt to explain disease on a rational basis. Because Hippocrates treated disease as a mass phenomenon as well as an individual occurrence, he has been called the "first epidemiologist." One of his most noteworthy contributions is the distinction between "endemic" diseases, which vary in prevalence from place to place, and "epidemic" diseases, which vary in prevalence over time. Hippocrates' writings are also the earliest in which there is a systematic attempt to relate the occurrence of disease to environmental factors. These relationships are examined in three of the books attributed to Hippocrates—*Epidemic I, Epidemic III*, and *On Airs, Waters and Places*.

Hippocrates' greatest contribution to epidemiology is one of approach. He carefully observed and recorded associations between certain diseases and such factors as geography, climate, diet, and living conditions. Lacking the statistical concepts so vital to modern epidemiology, he was only able to assess these observations intuitively. From a framework of observations, he built a theory of disease causation that was consistent with the philosophy of nature held by the leading Greek philosophers of his day.

The philosophy held that everything was composed of different combinations of particles that individually were too small to be seen. The hypothetical particles were known as "atoms." For this reason it was known as the *atomic theory*—a rather modern sounding term. However, unlike our modern atomic theory that identifies many different atoms, the ancient Greek atomic theory assumed only four kinds of atoms. There were atoms of earth, of air, of fire, and of water. Each atom possessed two of the four irreducible qualities of wetness, dryness, warmth, and coldness. Earth was cold and dry; air was hot and wet; water was cold and wet; and fire was hot and dry.

Hippocrates taught that the human body was composed of four (2) substances, which he called the four "humours"—blood, phlegm, yellow bile, and black bile. Each humour was made up of one type of atom. Thus, blood was made up of air and possessed the properties of being hot and wet. Likewise, phlegm was made up of water, yellow bile of fire, and black bile of earth. In health these four humours were in balance, with the body containing equal parts of each.

Consistent with the value that ancient Greek philosophers placed on moderation and balance, Hippocrates taught that illness resulted when an imbalance occurred in the humours. An excess of hot/wet blood, for instance, could produce fever, sweating, and diarrhea, while an excess of cold/dry black bile could cause chills and constipation.

In part, such an imbalance might be the result of diet. Spicy hot foods would stimulate the production of more of the hot humours—yellow bile or blood. Other foods might possess the properties of being cold, of being dry, or of being wet, and thus would stimulate the production of the humours with those properties. Some of the writings attributed to Hippocrates seem to place great emphasis on diet as a cause of disease, although others deny this possibility, giving diet a role in treatment but not in causation of disease.

More important than diet in Hippocrates' view was the influence of constitution. The term *constitution* is in some ways synonymous with (3) environment. It includes such obvious environmental factors as climate and major geographic features of the area (rivers, swamps, mountains). It also includes astrological influences and the influence of comets and meteors. The fiery trail of a comet or meteor was seen as obviously putting excess fire into the atmosphere, which could cause an epidemic of a yellow bile disease.

Hippocrates' approaches to treatment attempted to restore balance. Colds and other conditions associated with cold/wet phlegm were treated with hot spicy foods and applications of mustard or other irritants to the chest to produce a sensation of warmth. Fevers were treated by abstaining from food that might carry hot/wet air or hot/dry fire. There also were efforts to remove the excess humours. Excess blood was removed with leeches, by "cupping" (in which blood was drawn from cuts with a vacuum) or by simply opening a vein (or, sometimes, with disastrous results, an artery, as the distinction between veins and arteries was not yet known). Excess phlegm or black bile was sweated out in a steam bath or was eliminated by vomiting. Excess yellow bile or black bile was eliminated by high (or colonic) enemas.

Hippocrates still has a place in medical education. The Hippocratic Oath is, of course, both a medical tradition and a basis for medical ethics. As "the father of medicine," as well as "the first epidemiologist," Hippocrates is an important historical figure in the study of medicine. As recently as the first quarter of this century, however, the Hippocratic theory was still being taught in American medical schools not as history but as a valid theory of disease causation.

A great many elements of the Hippocratic theory have become a part of our common cultural heritage and thus of the way most of us think about disease. For instance, the widespread myth that chills and wet feet cause the common cold has its roots in the Hippocratic view that colds are due to an excess of phlegm (made up of the elements of earth and water). Likewise, the old saying, "Feed a cold and starve a fever," was a precept of Hippocratic medicine. In Puerto Rico and in New York City you can find traditional healers who practice "hot and cold therapy," a dietary therapy that is almost pure Hippocratic medicine. In many ways the Hippocratic tradition is still very much alive. Bloodletting remained a common medical practice until the late nineteenth century, colonic enemas continued to be a part of many physicians' practice in the early part of this century, and are still featured in many alternative health-care programs.

Hippocrates Revisited and Revised

The theories of Hippocrates were elaborated on more than half-a-century later by the Roman physician Galen. Born in the city of Pergamum in Asia Minor around 130 A.D., Galen began the study of medicine at an early age. At the age of 20 he began a sort of itinerant practice of medicine, wandering from place to place, apparently with no lasting professional or financial success. Eventually he became an army physician, which led to his becoming personal physician to the emperor Marcus Aurelius in 169 A.D. This privileged position allowed him ample time for research and writing. His literary output during this period was enormous. Although many of his manuscripts were destroyed in the year 192 and many more were lost over the ages since then, the texts that have survived amount to more than 90,000 words.

Galen's studies included the fields of anatomy and physiology, as well as theories of disease causation. His contributions to the field of physiology earned him the title "father of experimental physiology," while his writings on anatomy remained the accepted standard for 13 centuries. The dissection of human bodies, however, was as unacceptable a practice among the Romans as it was among the Greeks before them. Galen based his ideas of anatomy on what he had seen of wounded men in the army and in the gladiatorial arena, and on the dissection of animals—of the pig, the ape, the dog, and the ox. His anatomy showed the human breastbone to be segmented like that of an ape, the liver divided into many lobes like that of a hog, the uterus shaped in two long horns like that of a dog, the hip bones flared like those of an ox, and so on.

The manner in which he made his contributions to the understanding of disease causation made him the first "armchair epidemiologist." That is, he based his theories on the observations of others (especially of Hippocrates) rather than going out to make his own observations. Thus, his theory is basically an elaboration on Hippocrates' teachings.

In order to explain why some people become ill while others exposed to the same "constitution" do not, Galen added two new elements to Hippocrates' theory of the four humours and the constitution. These two new elements were knowm as *temperament* and *procatartic factors*. Procatartic factors referred to the influence of a person's way of life on the types of diseases from which he was likely to suffer. Slaves suffered from diseases quite different from those afflicting nobles; the disease experiences of merchants were quite different from those of soldiers or fishermen or farmers. In modern terms we might call these lifestyle factors or, even more appropriately, occupational factors.

In his concept of temperament, Galen disagreed with Hippocrates' teaching that human bodies are naturally composed of equal parts of the four humours. Instead he believed that in each person one humour predominated. This predominance of one humour or another was known as temperament. Of course, already being overendowed with one of the humours made the person especially vulnerable to the diseases associated with that humour.

An excess of each of the humours was associated not only with a particular disease vulnerability but also with a particular personality type. Persons with an inborn excess of blood, for instance, were said to have a sanguine temperament, characterized by a cheerful manner and optimistic outlook. The sanguine individual also possessed a typical appearance, with a robust red face and often with red hair as well—the blood showing through. Likewise, the phlegmatic person, oversupplied with cold watery phlegm, was passive and unexcitable, with dull, unexpressive features. An excess of black bile produced a melancholic temperament, prone to sadness and depression, and a thin, pale appearance. Yellow bile in excess produced a choleric personality that was easily aroused to anger—a hot temper and dry irritability from all that hot/dry fire in the yellow bile.

The Concept of Miasma

With the rise of Christianity the teaching of pagans such as Galen fell for a time into disfavor. Throughout most of Europe, demonic possession once again became the accepted explanation for all illnesses. The writings of many of the classic philosophers and scholars, including Galen, were preserved by Arab scholars following the rise of Christianity and the fall of the Roman Empire. Eventually, many of these "pagan" writings were reinterpreted by Christian scholars as part of the growing Christian theology, and were accepted by the Catholic Church. The accepted version of the writings of such pagans as Aristotle and Galen came to have almost scriptural authority.

The Hippocratic–Galenic theory as it survived into this era was far simpler and less sophisticated than its original sources. A complex theory was no competition for the demonic possession theory of disease with which it was to coexist for centuries. Influences such as climate and lifestyle were largely forgotten while the importance of comets and meteors as causes of epidemics remained prominent. Later physicians began to speak of "miasmas"—vapors rising from rotting refuse or stagnant water. These miasmas were seen as the means by which diseases were spread. When people breathed miasmas their humours were affected resulting in disease.

Preventive measures were centered on covering up or eliminating the miasmas. One slept with the windows closed in order to keep the night air out because it was believed that night air was particularly prone to carry miasmas (and also because demons were more likely to prowl at night). Herbs and incense were used to perfume the air, and to fill the nose and crowd out any miasmas. It was also believed that miasmas could be settled out of the air by loud noises; so that bells, gongs, and cannon fire were widely used as antiepidemic measures.

The miasma concept continues to dominate a great deal of popular thought about disease. As recently as two generations ago, many Americans wore asofoctida (or asofidity) bags around their necks in the winter to prevent colds and the flu (the bags contained asofetida and other pungent-smelling herbs). During World War II many allied military hospitals still burned incense to prevent infections. Today the public still spends money on camphor and menthol chest rubs, and on vapor-action cough drops.

Germ Theory

The successor to the Hippocratic–Galenic theory was the germ theory. The idea that living organisms might cause disease had been considered by physicians at least as far back as ancient Rome. Lucretius, Varro, and Columella all speculated on this possibility, but it wasn't until centuries later that <u>Fracastorius</u> developed a theory of disease based on this idea, and it was only in the late 19th century that it gained wide acceptance.

Fracastorius and the Concept of Contagion

Tradition holds that among the wonders of the New World brought back to Europe by Christopher Columbus, or at least by some of the seamen under his command, was a new disease. Faced with this new disease, the people of every European nation seemed compelled to blame the disease on another nation. The French called it "the Italian disease," the Poles called it "the disease of the Germans," the Russians called it "the Polish disease," and the English and the Italians called it "the French disease." One of the popularizers of the last of these nicknames was the 16th-century Italian physician and poet Hieronymus Fracastorius (1478–1553), author of the poem "Syphilidis, sive Morbi Gallici." In poetical form this work gave the disease its formal name <u>syphilis and summarized</u> the then current state of knowledge regarding the disease, its symptoms, and its treatment. It did this in the guise of a fable about a herdsman named Syphilos, who was the first victim of the disease, inflicted on him as punishment for blasphemy when he cursed the sun god for causing a drought that was killing his animals.

> He first wore buboes dreadful to the sight,
> First felt strange pains and sleepless past the night,
> From him the malady received its name.
> — *Fracastorius, Syphilidis, sive Morbi Gallici.*

Fracastorius was apparently a pen name, in latinized form, for Girolamo Fracastoro (or Fracastor), who practiced medicine in the Italian city-state of Verona. Apparently a very persuasive man, Fracastorius was able to popularize through his writings and personal contacts a radical new view of disease causation.

His theory was put forth in 1546 in a book entitled *De Res Contagiosa*. His theory was that disease was transferred from one person who has the disease to another person who then develops the disease. He called this transference *contagion* and argued that it occurred through the conveyance of disease by tiny imperceptible particles, which he called *seminaria contagium*—seeds (or germs) of contagion.

Fracastorius distinguished three types of contagion. The basic type was spread by direct contact only. In the second type, the germs of contagion were conveyed person-to-person by what he called fomes— "clothing, wooden objects, and things of that sort, which though not themselves corrupted, can, nevertheless, preserve the original germs of the contagion and infect by means of these—which a modern epidemiologist would call fomites. Thirdly, there were contagions that could infect "at a distance."

One important person who was convinced by Fracastorius of the merits of his theory was Pope Paul III. It is as a result of Pope Paul's belief in the theory of contagion that the Council of Trent was held in Bologna, Italy instead of in Trent, France (an important event in the history of the church). The presence of contagious disease in Trent (apparently syphilis among the prostitutes of Trent) was recognized by the Pope as a threat to the church leaders and so he transferred the council to Bologna where the conditions did not exist. Such support for the theory did not outlive Fracastorius. Following his death, the concept of contagion was largely forgotten for the next 200 years.

The concept of quarantine—the exclusion or isolation of persons suffering from certain diseases—was not forgotten. Although quarantine continued to be practiced, acceptance of the practice was based as much on the demonic and miasma concepts of disease as on any concept of contagion.

In the late 18th century, the English physician John Hoygarth used true epidemiologic methods in studying the spread of fever within families from the first diseased family member. From the patterns of distribution that he found, he inferred that different diseases had different incubation or latent periods during which infection is present but symptoms have not developed. In 1774 he proposed that instead of quarantining fever victims within their own homes, they should be isolated in "spacious airy, separate apartments," within a special "fever ward" of a hospital. Nine years later, he established the first such ward in the attic of the infirmary in the city of Chester. The success of the Chester "fever ward" soon led to the establishment of similar units in Manchester, Liverpool, and other cities, and gave momentum to the rise of a contagion-centered theory of disease—germ theory.

The Discovery of Microorganisms

One barrier to acceptance of the concept of contagion had been the notion of invisible particles or of living things too small to be seen. Invisible miasmas were easy enough to believe in; everyone knew that you can't see an odor. But, obviously, no one had ever seen an invisible particle or an invisible organism.

A retired Dutch drape-maker by the name of Anton van Leeuwenhoek (1632–1723) provided the answer to this objection. The writings of Galileo, banned in most of Europe, were readily available in the tiny libertarian country of Holland. Astronomy and telescopes were very much in fashion as gentlemen's hobbies in the Holland of van Leeuwenhoek's time. He was one of the first to adapt the principle of the telescope to the task of examining very small things close up instead of examining very big things far away. In brief, he invented the microscope.

Peering through his simple microscope, van Leeuwenhoek discovered tiny living things in a drop of water. These tiny organisms, which he called "animalcules," were soon recognized as the invisible living things in the contagion concept. The connection was made by some but it was not yet germ theory's day.

"Clean Hands May Carry the Disease"

Childbirth was long one of the major causes of death. The principal reason for this was puerperal fever, or childbirth fever, which struck females a few hours to a few days after giving birth to a child. High fever, weak rapid pulse, and abdominal pain often led to the death of the female. Puerperal fever became increasingly common as more women began having their babies delivered in a maternity hospital (or "lying-in hospital"). Epidemics of puerperal fever occurred in these hospitals and were blamed on miasmas associated with the weather. It is reported that in the year 1776 the weather was such that not one woman survived childbirth in the city of Lombardy.

In 1845, Oliver Wendell Holmes, a physician better known as a literary figure and father of a Supreme Court Justice, wrote a paper called "The Contagiousness of Puerperal Fever." In this paper Holmes argued that puerperal fever was an infection transmitted from one patient to another by the physician or midwife. The reaction to this radical view ranged from indifference to outrage.

In a later paper entitled "Puerperal Fever as a Private Pestilence," Holmes replied to his critics. In it he referred to the work of a physician named "Senderein," who had lessened the mortality due to the disease by washing his hands with chloride of lime. He replied to the criticisms of a Dr. Meigs, who had resented the suggestion that physicians had dirty hands, and cited the case of a Dr. Simpson who though an "eminent gentleman" (and thus presumably incapable of having dirty hands) had nevertheless had a number of cases of puerperal fever among the women he had assisted in childbirth. Holmes replied that if that was true, then "it follows that a gentleman with clean hands may carry the disease." Once the initial furor over these two papers had died down, the medical community soon forgot all about Holmes' unpleasant idea.

The "Dr. Senderein" referred to by Holmes was actually Ignaz Semmelweis (1818–1865). Semmelweis was a Hungarian who began studying law at the University of Vienna but switched to medicine and eventually specialized in, and revolutionized the field of, obstetrics. After graduation he obtained a position at the University of Vienna's maternity hospital. He was in charge of the hospital's First Division in which babies were delivered by medical students. In the Second Division midwife students delivered the babies.

Semmelweis discovered that over a 60-year period the death rate due to puerperal fever in the First Division ranged from 68 to 158 deaths per 1,000 births with an average of 99 deaths per 1,000 births. In the Second Division over the same period the death rate from puerperal fever overaged 33 per 1,000 births. It was this substantial difference between the death rates of the two populations of patients that set him to search for a cause.

Semmelweis was able to quickly dismiss such possible explanations of the difference as miasmas arising from dirty laundry or accumulating due to poor ventilation. The condition of laundry and ventilation in both divisions were equally poor. Likewise, he concluded that poor diet could not be the cause of the difference because the food was the same in both divisions.

One theory that had been proposed was that the high rate of puerperal fever was caused by embarrassment. The modesty of the women in the First Division, it was suggested, had been outraged by having male physicians care for them during childbirth. Semmelweis rejected this theory, in part because most of his patients did not seem to be particularly modest. More convincingly, he pointed out that women of the upper classes who were usually attended to by male physicians when in labor did not experience a high rate of puerperal fever. Yet another suggestion was that the high rate was caused by fear. Women were afraid of being cared for in the First Division and this fear, it was argued, caused them to develop puerperal fever. The circularity of this logic was obvious to Semmelweis. The women were afraid of the First Division because of the high death rate, so their fears could not have caused the high death rate.

Semmelweis found that the only difference between the two divisions was who delivered the babies. He looked for differences between the ways that medical students and midwife students delivered babies and found none—they were, after all, being trained by the same teachers. The one difference (aside from sex) that he did find between the medical students and the midwife students was in the way they spent their time between deliveries. When not delivering babies, the midwife students made tea, gossiped, and knitted. Between births the medical students dissected cadavers—dead bodies.

At about the same time that Semmelweis made the above observation, one of his colleagues, Dr. Kolletschka, died. Dr. Kolletschka's finger had been cut when a student's scalpel slipped while they were dissecting a body. He died as a result of this slight wound. Semmelweis noted that the symptoms of Dr. Kolletschka's fatal illness were the same as those of puerperal fever. The two observations led him to conclude that puerperal fever was at such a high rate in the First Division because of something the medical students got on their hands while dissecting the unrefrigerated bodies. With this in mind, he ordered all of his medical students to wash their hands in a solution of chloride of lime before seeing any patients. At that time the puerperal fever death rate in the First Division was 120 per 1,000 births. In the 7 months after his hand-washing rule went into effect, the rate was 12 deaths per 1,000 births—the first time in the history of the hospital that the death rate in the First Division was lower than that in the Second. Also for the first time ever there were 2 months in which no patients in the First Division died.

This great contribution resulted in Semmelweis being suspended from his position for 6 months and, subsequently, being subjected to a variety of harassments. He left Vienna abruptly and returned to his home in Budapest, where he became head of the maternity hospital and wrote a book on his findings on puerperal fever. His theory was regarded by many of his colleagues as evidence of insanity. Eventually, he was sent back to Vienna as a mental patient. When examined at the mental hospital, it was discovered that he had a cut on his finger that had probably resulted during one of his last operations. He died of the fever he had first recognized as being same thing as puerperal fever. Unlike Fracastorius, Semmelweis' ideas did live on after him, although acceptance was slow.

"Germ Theory Achieves Dominance"

Germ theory came to be the dominant theory of disease under the leadership of Louis Pasteur (1827–1912). It is a surprise to many to discover that Pasteur was not a physician. He was in fact a chemist whose work had originally centered on the study of crystals. He had written his dissertation on two forms of tartaric acid, and this led naturally to the study of wine because tartaric acid is one of the naturally occurring substances that gives wine its flavor. Pasteur's attention was drawn to the diseases of wine—a problem of serious importance to the French economy of his time.

For centuries it had been known that if grapes were crushed the juice would naturally ferment forming alcohol and turning the grape juice into wine. No one knew how or why this natural process took place, nor why the process stopped as automatically as it started. About 15 percent of the juice would be turned into alcohol but no more. Equally, it was not known why the process went bad in diseased wine. But it was known that in some batches the juice putrified producing a bitter, ropy wine. This unpredictable sickness could wipe out a single batch or an entire vintage. The person who could prevent sick batches of wine could save the wine industry from periodic losses that were at times disastrous. If that person could learn how to get the fermentation process to continue beyond its natural limit, then that person would possess knowledge worth a fortune. Pasteur set out to be that person.

Pasteur discovered that fermentation was a result of the growth of yeast in the grape juice. The yeasts grew naturally in small amounts on the skin of the grape. When the grape was crushed the yeasts reached the sugar-rich juice and multiplied prolifically. Each of the microscopic yeast organisms consumed sugar from the juice and excreted alcohol as a waste product. Any organism's waste products are poisonous to that organism when they are in a high enough concentration. When the level of alcohol in wine rises to about 15 percent, the yeasts die off having been poisoned by the rising concentration of their own excrement. Thus Pasteur, in discovering how fermentation took place, had also learned that it could not be made to continue beyond its natural stopping point. He was able, however, to learn the cause and means of prevention for sick wine. Diseased wine, he found, contained bacteria that had replaced the yeasts that should have reproduced in the juice. He found that this could be prevented by heating the grape juice to a temperature high enough to kill off any organisms in it but not high enough to damage the juice. This process came to be known as *pasteurization*. Once the grape juice was pasteurized the winemaker could add yeast from a good batch of wine to assure that the healthy fermentation process took place. Later, when it was learned that milk was commonly a source of infection with the germs of tuberculosis, typhoid, and other diseases, pasteurization of milk became an important public health measure.

Pasteur next turned his attention to a disease that was of major economic importance. The silk industry, one of France's leading industries at that time, was threatened by an epidemic that could have destroyed the industry. Pasteur was able to identify two separate infections that were attacking the silkworms and developed a preventive for each. Out of gratitude for his contributions to two of France's major industries, the French government provided Pasteur with a house, a laboratory, and a pension. This left Pasteur free to pursue his interests without worrying about financial support. He continued his researches into disease, studying anthrax and chicken cholera.

It was in the course of his studies of chicken cholera that Pasteur made a discovery of far-reaching significance. He had isolated the bacteria that is the agent of chicken cholera. He grew this bacteria in a broth that had to be renewed periodically or the bacteria would be poisoned by their own waste products (like the yeast in wine). Pasteur renewed his cultures of the bacteria by putting a few drops of the old broth (containing the bacteria) into the fresh broth. A few drops of this broth placed on bread and fed to a chicken invariably resulted in the chicken developing chicken cholera and dying. Through an oversight, Pasteur let some of his broth go longer than usual without being renewed. When he fed this broth to some chickens, the became sick but did not die. Furthermore, when he later fed the chickens a full-strength bacterial broth, they did not become ill. They had acquired an immunity to chicken cholera by overcoming the infection with the bacteria from the weakened culture. Thus, Pasteur had discovered the principle of *bacterial vaccination.* He was to apply this principle in developing vaccines for a number of important diseases. The greatest impact was to result from his work on rabies.

Although more common in the 19th century than today, rabies was not one of the leading causes of death at the time. It was more feared than many of the biggest killers. With other diseases there was always the possibility of recovery but rabies was always fatal. To be bitten by a rabid animal was a sure sentence of death—and an extremely painful death. No medical treatment could save the life of a rabies victim or relieve the pain.

Through a lengthy series of experiments, Pasteur was able to establish that the infectious organism for rabies was located in the nervous systems of rabid animals. He was not, however, able to isolate the organism. He could not see the organism under a microscope. He could extract the organism in a culture but when he tried to filter out the organism it passed right through the filter. As a result he called the organism a filtrable virus, a name that means a living thing able to pass through a filter.

Pasteur was able, nevertheless, to develop a vaccine for rabies. He infected rabbits with rabies and then, when they died, removed their spinal cords. He weakened the virus by drying the spinal cords and then ground up this material to make his vaccine. He not only developed a normal vaccine to protect persons or animals against becoming infected with rabies, but also developed the Pasteur prophylaxis, which could be administered to persons who had already been infected with rabies. When a person was infected with rabies, the first symptoms did not develop until 3 weeks or more later. Immunity could be established in less time with a series of injections of the Pasteur prophylaxis. In 1885, Pasteur administered his prophylaxis to Joseph Meister, a 9-year-old boy who had been bitten in fourteen places by a rabid dog. The boy did not develop rabies. Soon afterwards, Pasteur administered the treatment to a 14-year-old shepherd boy named Berger Gupile, who had become a hero by struggling with a rabid dog to prevent it from biting some younger children. Again the prophylaxis saved the boy from developing the fatal disease. As word of these successes reached the public, Pasteur became an international celebrity. This victory of germ theory over a particularly feared disease gave a tremendous boost to public acceptance of germ theory.

If Pasteur is the father of germ theory, then Robert Koch must be its godfather. Koch was a German biologist whose many contributions include the discovery of the germs of tuberculosis (TB) and cholera, and the development of the tuberculin skin test for TB. His most important contribution, however, was a set of four logical steps, known as "Koch's Postulates," to establish a causal relationship between a microorganism and a disease. In an 1882 paper in which Koch first announced his discovery of the tubercle bacillus, he states the postulates in a crude

form as a refutation to the argument made by some miasma theorists—
that the germs he had found were symptoms of tuberculosis rather than
the cause of it. Eight years later he stated them in their fully developed
form, as follows:

> If one can now, however, prove: first, that the parasite in each
> individual case of the disease in question can be found and indeed under
> conditions which correspond to the pathologic changes and the clinical
> course of the disease; second, that it does not occur in any other disease as
> a chance and nonpathogenic parasite; and third, that it is capable of being
> isolated... from the body and in pure cultures sufficiently often trans-
> formed in order to cause the disease anew; then it can no longer be a
> random accident of the disease, but between the parasite and the disease
> can be conceived no relation except that the parasite is the cause of the
> disease. (Koch, 1890, p. 35).

The adoption of such strict and clearly logical standards for establishing causation greatly strengthened the case for germ theory. The
postulates are entirely consistent with germ theory's contention that
every disease is caused by a germ and by that germ alone. The possibility
that infection with a germ might not cause disease in every instance was
as alien to the germ theorists' assumptions as was noninfectious
disease.

Koch, however, was to run into problems with the application of his
own postulates to his isolation of the cholera bacillus. He had no
difficulty in meeting the requirements of the first three postulates:
present in all cases and at all stages, not present in other diseases, and
isolated from the body in pure cultures. But he could not satisfy, the
fourth postulate (often referred to as "experimental disease") by
causing the disease anew with that culture. In the first place, he
encountered this difficulty because the cholera bacillus is what is
known as an obligate parasite—one that can live as a parasite only in a
single species of animal—in man. It was impossible, therefore, for
Koch to produce the disease in any laboratory animal. It was soon
demonstrated, however, that the problem went beyond the inability
to produce the disease in other animals. The German hygienist Max
von Petenkoffer, and the French biologist and nutritionist Elie
Metchnikoff, both opponents of germ theory, repeatedly drank glasses
of cultures isolated from fatal cases of cholera without suffering any
ill effects. In fact, no one has ever succeeded in producing anything
more than mild diarrhea in volunteers given even massive amounts
of the cholera bacillus.

Koch developed tuberculin in his search for a vaccine against tuberculosis. Although tuberculin proved to be ineffective as a vaccine, it produced an allergic reaction in persons who were infected with the tubercle bacillus. This provided the basis for wide use of the TB skin test in screening for tuberculosis. When Koch injected himself with tuberculin he experienced a very severe allergic reaction, indicating that he himself had a massive TB infection even though he never suffered the disease. This was one more situation incompatible with germ theory's simplistic equation of infection with disease.

In the following chapter we will discuss how classic epidemiologic theory arose, first as a refinement of germ theory, and eventually as its replacement.

Recommended Reading _____

Dubos, R. (1959). *Mirage of health.* Garden City, NY: Doubleday and Company. [Especially useful are Chapters 4 and 5.]

Haggard, H. W. (1929). *Devils, drugs and doctors.* New York: Harper and Brothers. [Especially Chapters 4 (regarding Semmelweis), 16 (Pasteur), and 17 (Hippocrates and Galen).]

Rosen, G. (1958). *A history of public health.* New York: MD Publications.

Winslow, C. E. A. (1923). *The evolution and significance of the modern public health campaign.* New Haven: Yale University Press. Reprinted in 1984 by the *Journal of Public Health Policy Inc.,* South Burlington, VT.

CHAPTER 2

Classic Epidemiologic Theory

As the inadequacies of germ theory became increasingly evident, epidemiologists began to rethink the causation of disease. This new and broader formulation was perhaps most clearly stated by Theobald Smith in his 1934 book, *Parasitism and Disease*. Concerning himself only with the infectious diseases, Smith explained disease as an instance of parasitism, in which the infectious agent lives in or on the human host. He saw disease as the result of forces within a dynamic system consisting of the agent of infection, the host, and the environment— which came to be known as the *epidemiologic triad.*

In terms of this model, patterns of disease depend on factors that determine the probability of contact between an infectious agent and a susceptible host. The route by which the agent is shed by an ill host, the length of time over which it is shed, the climatic conditions surrounding the host, and the presence of alternate nonhuman hosts that may serve as a continuing reservoir of infection all play a part in determining whether a host will be exposed to infection. The availability of susceptible hosts depends on population density and mobility, community vaccination status, and extent and degree of immunity from previous infections with the same or related agents.

Eventually, the concept of agent was generalized beyond infectious agents. Many epidemiologists found that this model was applicable to noninfectious diseases as well as those with infectious agents. The term *agent* had to be reconceptualized beyond infectious organisms. In terms of this broader conceptualization, the agent is the one factor that *must* be present for the disease to occur (as the smallpox virus, for example, must be present for a case of smallpox to occur). In the terms of formal logic, an agent is a necessary but not sufficient cause of a disease; that is, a particular disease cannot occur without the agent even though the presence of the agent does not, by itself, guarantee that the disease will occur.

Types of Agents

We can define an agent as an organism, substance, or force whose relative presence or relative absence is necessary for a particular disease process to occur. In this definition you will see that one further element has entered the concept of agent. In some diseases it is the lack of some organism, substance, or force that makes the disease process possible. In the following descriptions of the types of agents it can be seen that there are those of each type that make disease possible through their presence or excess, and those that make disease possible through their absence or deficiency.

Living Organisms

The many varieties of infectious agents—of viruses, bacteria, amoebas, and so on—are the agents first identified by the germ theorists. To this may be added a variety of external parasites, such as lice (for pediculosis), mites (for scabies), or fungi (for athlete's foot). There is also a form of diarrhea that results in persons whose "intestinal flora" (the bacteria normally found in plentiful quantity in the bowel) has been killed off by antibiotics or radiation.

Nutritive Elements

We are most familiar with nutrients as agents in instances where it is their relative absence that is necessary for the disease process to occur. Lind's (1753) demonstration that citrus fruits are a preventive of scurvy[1] is one of the first discoveries of a disease with a nutritive element as its agent. Scurvy was finally found to be due to a lack of

---

[1] Discussed in Chapter 11.

vitamin C (ascorbic acid). Since that time there have been a whole range of vitamin deficiency diseases identified. More recently, a dietary deficiency of protein has been identified as the agent of kwashiorkor. On the other hand, saturated fats may be the agent of arteriosclerosis (hardening of the arteries). Some epidemiologists have speculated that sodium (especially in the form of salt) might be the agent of hypertension (high blood pressure), but this hypothesis is increasingly in doubt. If obesity can be regarded as a disease, then calories in general might be regarded as its agent.

Exogenous Chemicals

The term *exogenous chemicals* refers to those chemicals (other than nutrients) affecting the body that originate outside the body. Technically, this term is identical to the definition of a drug (Duncan & Gold, 1982) but it is used here to convey a broader sense than that in which the term drug is ordinarily used. Alcohol is the agent of alcoholism as nicotine is the agent of tobacco addiction. The range of other exogenous chemical agents extends over the entire scope of irritants, poisons, and allergens arising outside the host—from arsenic to ragweed pollen. Fox, Hall, and Elveback (1970) muse on whether the agent of drowning is water (too much) or air (too little) in the lungs of the host.

Endogenous Chemicals

The human body itself gives rise to chemicals that may act as agents. These may be abnormal products, such as those that arise from the breakdown of tissue in extensive burns. More often they are normal bodily products that are in relative excess or deficiency. Excesses or deficiencies in the production of various hormones serve as the agents for a number of diseases. For example, if pituitary growth hormone is oversecreted during childhood it is the agent of giantism, and when undersecreted it is the agent of dwarfism; in adulthood oversecretion of growth hormone is the agent of acromegaly, a disfiguring disorder in which the bones and cartilage of the face, hands, and feet resume growth, becoming greatly enlarged. An excess of uric acid is the agent of gout, a form of arthritis in which crystals of uric acid are deposited in joints, usually of the hands or feet.

Genetic Traits

A number of diseases have been identified as having a gene or combination of genes as their agent. These range from the very common, such as alopecia (pattern baldness), through the less than rare, such as diabetes, to the rare, such as Tay-Sachs disease or hemophilia. Some others, such as Down's syndrome (mongolism), have as their agent some structural abnormality of the chromosomes.

Psychological Factors and Stress

These are undoubtedly the most speculated on but least understood of the agents. It can, for instance, be argued that stress *or* excessive gastric acid (an endogenous chemical) is the agent of stomach ulcers. Similar ambiguity is to be encountered with other possible psychic agents.

Physical Forces

Most of us have experienced sunburn for which the agent is ultraviolet light. Likewise, the agent of radiation sickness is ionizing radiation. The agent for fractures is mechanical force (including that resulting from gravity) against a bone. The agent of caisson disease or "the bends" is excessive atmospheric pressure—nitrogen becomes soluble in the blood of divers operating under high air pressure for deep dives and forms bubbles in their blood if they return to normal pressure too soon. Low atmospheric pressure, on the other hand, is the agent for altitude sickness.

Characteristics of Infectious Agents

Infectious agents vary in their inherent ability to infect and produce disease in a host. The ability of an infectious organism to invade and multiply in a host is known as *infectivity*. This is usually measured by the *secondary attack rate*, which is:

$$\frac{\text{Number of exposed hosts developing disease within the maximum incubation period after exposure}}{\text{Total number of susceptible exposed hosts}} \times 100$$

For a given infectious agent, of course, this may vary greatly from one species of host to another or, within one host species, with the manner of transmission or differing host characteristics.

Pathogenicity refers to the ability of an agent to produce disease in an infected host. This may be measured by calculating:

$$\frac{\text{Number of cases of disease}}{\text{Total number infected}} \times 100$$

This varies from highly pathogenic agents, such as those of rabies, smallpox, measles, and chickenpox, which produce illness in virtually every infected host to, for instance, poliovirus, which produces illness only once in every 300–1,000 infections.

Although the term *virulence* is commonly used by physicians as a synonym for pathogenicity, it really means the ability of an infectious agent to produce severe illness in diseased hosts. Severe illness is a difficult concept to define in a way that can be concretely applied to all diseases. For this reason, it has become accepted practice to use the case fatality rate as a proxy measure[2] for virulence. The case fatality rate is:

$$\frac{\begin{array}{c}\text{Number of deaths due to a given disease}\\\text{during a specified period of time}\end{array}}{\begin{array}{c}\text{Number of cases of that disease}\\\text{occurring in the same period of time}\end{array}} \times 100$$

Virulence varies from diseases such as chickenpox, rubella, or the common cold, which almost never produce any form of severe illness to such extremely virulent diseases as rabies—a fatal illness—or acquired immunodeficiency syndrome (AIDS)—which results in death in 80 percent of all cases within 2 years after diagnosis. Smallpox, which is fatal in 20–40 percent of all cases, may seem minor in comparison to rabies and AIDS but is highly virulent compared to most human diseases.

Although these concepts developed specifically with reference to infectious agents, they have some applicability to other types of agents. They help to emphasize the point that while the agent is necessary for

---

[2]A proxy measure does not actually measure the hard-to-measure concept you wish to measure, but instead measures a second more easily measured concept that parallels the one you wish to measure. This gives an estimate of the first concept but not a true measure of it.

the disease to occur it is not sufficient. As Rene Dubos (1965), has stated, "Throughout nature, infection without disease is the rule rather than the exception" (p. 190).

Vectors of Transmission

Many agents are transmitted from host to host by blood-sucking insects. Malaria, yellow fever, and encephalitis are conveyed from host to host by mosquitoes. Plague and murine typhus are both conveyed by rat fleas. Rocky Mountain spotted fever is carried by ticks. The term *vector* was coined for such blood-sucking insects as carriers of infection.

Other animals also convey agents from host-to-host. Epidemic typhus, for instance, is carried by the human body louse. Rabies is carried by the bite of an infected animal. These were sometimes referred to as vectors, although they are not blood-sucking insects. Many agents may be carried on the feet of flies whose taste buds are located in the soles of their feet, and who therefore taste possible food by walking on it.

Agents may also be conveyed from one host to another via non-living items. These nonliving carriers have been called *vehicles* or *mechanical vectors.* Included would be hypodermics shared by drug addicts, which can convey serum hepatitis or AIDS. Intimate personal items, such as handkerchiefs, toothbrushes, or tobacco pipes, which are not normally shared between people and which can carry agents from person to person when they are shared, are called *fomites* by epidemiologists.

The distinctions between vectors, vehicles, and fomites seem to have been treated with less importance in recent years. The term *vector* is increasingly used for all means by which agents may be conveyed from one host to another. It has been broadened by some theorists far beyond any of these original concepts and has even been applied by some epidemiologists (c.f. Justice & Duncan, 1975; Justice & Justice, 1976) to abstract concepts that may bring psychic agents to bear on potential hosts.

Host Factors

Hosts differ in their exposure to agents and in the likelihood of their developing a disease in response to the agent. They vary in the state of their natural defenses against disease as well as in the behaviors that may expose them to agents.

Immunity and Immunologic Responses

Specific immunity to infectious disease is usually the result of the body's production of substances known as antibodies. These antibodies are present in the blood, tissue fluids, and often the mucous secretions of the immune host. The immunity possessed by a host is classified on the one hand as being active or passive and on the other hand as being natural or artificial.

Active immunity means that the host is producing its own antibodies. Natural active immunity (or naturally acquired active immunity) is the result of having previously had and recovered from a case of the disease. Artificial (or artificially acquired) active immunity is the result of vaccination.

Passive immunity means that the host possesses antibodies but is not capable of producing its own new antibodies when the old ones "wear out" with age. Newborn infants possess natural passive immunity to the diseases that their mothers are immune to, due to the passage through the placenta of antibodies from the mother's blood to the fetus' blood. In breast-fed infants the mother continues to replenish the infants' natural passive immunity by transmitting antibodies through her milk. Passive immunity may also be artificially induced by injecting antibody material acquired from an actively immune host. Gamma globulin, the antibody-containing fraction of pooled adult human blood plasma, is used for short-term protection against infectious hepatitis and measles. Likewise, antibodies from horses (or sometimes other animals) are used to provide temporary immunity to tetanus or rabies.

Host Behavior

The behavior of a potential host determines in large part the likelihood of exposure to agents or the degree of susceptibility to disease. The best known systematic examination of this broad area is the well-known work of Belloc and Breslow (1972). They identified five health habits that were highly associated with lower death rates and better health status. These five health habits were: sleeping 7–8 hours per night, exercising moderately several times per week, maintaining normal weight, not smoking, and drinking either in moderation or not at all.

Environmental Factors ─────────────────────────────

Environmental factors affect both the exposure of potential hosts to agents and the ability of the hosts to maintain high levels of resistance. The environment may be thought of as being comprised of three broad areas: the physical, which includes the geographic, geologic, and climatic features of the environment; the biological, which includes all the living creatures in the environment; and the social, which includes social institutions, cultural norms, and economic features of the environment.

Physical Environment

Geographic features may influence the occurrence of disease. Geographic features such as mountain ranges, rivers, or deserts may constitute natural boundaries limiting the spread of disease agents or their vectors. On the other hand, trade routes provided by roads, rivers, or mountain passes may also constitute the routes along which diseases spread from place to place. Geographic features may also provide ideal circumstances for a concentration of disease agents or vectors. For instance, malaria, yellow fever, and encephalitis are more common in low-lying, swampy areas that provide an ideal home for the mosquitoes that carry the agent.

Climate and geography are often related in their effects on the distribution of disease. Epidemic typhus, for example, is found only in temperate zones and high altitude areas of the subtropics, whereas murine typhus is common in the lowlands of the tropics and subtropics. The cooler climate in which epidemic typhus is found encourages the wearing of many clothes. That, along with infrequent laundering, favors the human body louse that spreads the infection of epidemic typhus. The warm climate of the tropical and subtropical lowlands discourages wearing many clothes and lice infestation but favors an abundance of rats, the fleas of which carry the agent of murine typhus.

Geologic formations determine the ability of soil to hold and purify water, the availability and types of fuel and mineral deposits, and the ability of soils to support crops. These features may have great impact on disease patterns in the population.

Biological Environment

The distribution of disease is often affected by the plentifulness of vectors or alternate hosts in the environment. The role of such vectors

as rat fleas and mosquitoes has already been noted. Rabies is conveyed
to humans by contact with rabid animals. Because rabies is common
among skunks, nearness to a large skunk population increases the risk
of rabies. Encephalitis infection is common among birds and is carried
from bird to bird by mosquitoes. When the bird population is reduced by
a bad winter, for instance, the mosquitoes that normally prey on birds
seek nourishment elsewhere, biting people and conveying the infection
to them.

Social Environment

Population density relates to the adequacy of food, water, and other
resources. The age distribution within a population has major impact
on the disease experiences of that population. A youthful population
will suffer higher rates of infectious diseases and traumatic injuries,
while an older population will suffer more from degenerative and other
chronic diseases.

Many of the host behaviors that affect exposure and susceptibility to
disease are culturally patterned. For instance, the dietary pattern and
food-handling practices within a society influence not only the
exposure to nutritive elements as agents but also exogenous chemicals
and living agents with which foods may become contaminated. Patterns
of personal hygiene and of waste disposal have major effects on the
exposure of the population to many agents.

The same is true of norms for personal contact. For instance, in our
society epidemics of the parasitic disease scabies, which is readily
transmitted through hand-holding, is seen mostly in preschool and
elementary school children who often hold hands. In Arab societies it is
not uncommon for men to hold hands while walking together—as a
result, scabies epidemics often extend to the adult population. The
relevance to venereal diseases is even more obvious.

Recommended Readings _____

Brander, G. C., & Ellis, P. R. (1977). *The control of disease.* London: Bailliere
    Tindall.
Justice, B., & Justice, R. (1976). *The abusing family.* New York: Human Science
    Press.
Rogers, P. (1977). *Everyday problems in public health.* Philadelphia: F. A. Davis
    Company.

CHAPTER 3

Multicausality and Webs of Causation

Germ theory suffered the weakness of being a single cause theory. All diseases were presumed to be caused by germs and by germs alone—one species of germ per disease. When infection with, for instance, the cholera germ occurred, then the disease cholera should surely follow. The repeated proof that this was not true has not ended the tendency of most people to seek an understanding of disease in terms of a single cause.

When most people think of the cause of disease, they think in terms of a single cause. Evidence that smoking causes lung cancer is countered with the tale of Uncle Charlie, who smoked two packs a day and died at 97 without a sign of cancer. Even more compelling is the case of cousin Sue, who died of lung cancer despite the fact that she never smoked a cigarette in her life. In each case, smoking is being assessed as a single and certain cause of cancer, when it is, in fact, only one of a set of interrelated factors that together can cause cancer.

The classic epidemiologic triad of host, agent, and environment provides a better model for understanding the complex realities of disease causation. This model, however, developed almost entirely as a model for the understanding of infectious diseases. The centrality of the concept of agent is in many ways a carryover from germ theory. In the triad model, the single element of the agent is represented as if it were equal in importance to the variety of relevant factors in the host and the multitude of environmental influences. The actual findings of epidemiology in the study of a vast array of diseases have not supported this exaggerated weighting given to the agent as a cause of disease.

During the present century, medical and social progress have reduced the impact of infectious diseases on society and have increased public health concern with the chronic diseases. Difficulties have been encountered in applying the concept of agent to many of the chronic diseases. In fact, it often has seemed more like an intellectual game than a useful pursuit, to try to identify a single factor without which the particular disease under study could not occur.

The nature of this problem may be illustrated by reference to an attempt to develop a causal model of child abuse in terms of host-agent-environment-vector (Justice & Duncan, 1975, 1977; Justice & Justice, 1976). Viewing child abuse as a disorder within the parent dyad or parent (host), what element must always be present (or always be deficient) in order for child abuse to occur? The answer given by this model is that the child is the agent of child abuse. Obviously, child abuse cannot occur without a child—but this is an extension of the term agent beyond its original usage.

In seeking a model that better expresses the complex reality of multicausality, some epidemiologists began thinking in terms of chains of causation. In a chain of causation we looked at a causal event, then at the antecedents of that event, then at the antecedents of the antecedent, and so on. For instance, we note that a person developed a febrile illness known as leptospirosis after becoming infected with *Leptospira interrogans*; this organism entered through a cut finger while the person was emptying a cat litter box; this was possible because the litter was contaminated with *Leptospira*; this was because the cat had leptospirosis—a common disease of cats—and was shedding the infectious organism in its urine. The chain of causation is thus: Infected cat → contaminated urine → contaminated litter → infected cut → leptospirosis in host.

Such chains, however, left much out. For instance, this chain of events would not have occurred if the host had not had a cut finger. It would not have occurred if the host had worn rubber gloves to change the litter box. It might not have occurred if there had been a bandage on the cut. It probably would not have occurred if the host had promptly washed after changing the litter box. It would not have occurred if the host had an immunity due to a prior case of the same type of leptospirosis or vaccination against that type of leptospirosis. It would not have occurred if the cat had been placed in isolation at a veterinary clinic until it was cured. It would not have occurred if the cat had been immunized against leptospirosis. And so forth.

Another example of a chain of causation is the "diet–heart hypo-thesis" (DHH) as described by Sherwin (1978). As hypothesized in this chain, a diet high in saturated fat and cholesterol leads to high blood lipids, which lead to atherosclerosis (coronary artery disease), which leads to coronary heart disease and the clinical event of a myocardial infarct (heart attack). This simple chain, however, leaves out many important elements. Sherwin notes, for instance, that the link between diet and elevated blood lipids is also influenced by genetic factors and emotional stress. The link between high blood lipids and atheroscle-rosis is also promoted by genetic factors, aging, hypertension, smoking, stress, and low blood levels of the protective high-density-lipoprotein cholesterol (HDL). Genetics, smoking, and stress again contribute to the link between atherosclerosis and coronary heart disease, as does the presence of free-floating blood clots (emboli), which can block an artery already constricted by atherosclerosis. Adequate representation of all of these additional elements requires a more complex model than the simple chain of causation. An expanded version of this chain of causation is shown in Figure 3.1.

MacMahon, Pugh, and Ipsen (1960) recognized that chains of causa-tion suffered from "the defect of oversimplification" and proposed a new model that they called a "web of causation." Their first attempt at such a chain or web was to explain the occurrence of icterus (or jaundice) among some patients being treated for syphilis (see Figure 3.2). Of this expanded chain of causation they state:

> When it is considered that only a few of the major components are shown, that these are indicated as broad classes of events rather than as the multiple minor events comprising each class, that each component shown is itself the result of a complex genealogy of antecedents, and that the myriad of effects of these components other than those contributing to the development of icterus are not shown, then the "chains" of causation become difficult to elucidate and the whole genealogy might be thought of more appropriately as a web, which in its complexity and origins lies quite beyond our understanding. Fortunately, to effect preventive measures, it is not necessary to understand causal mechanisms in their entirety. (p. 18)

In an attempt to more fully represent the "genealogy" of the disease and its causes, in a web of causation not only is the disease seen as having multiple causes, but each of these causes is seen as being an effect that resulted from multiple causes, each of which is an effect resultant to multiple causes, and so on. Each arrow on a web of

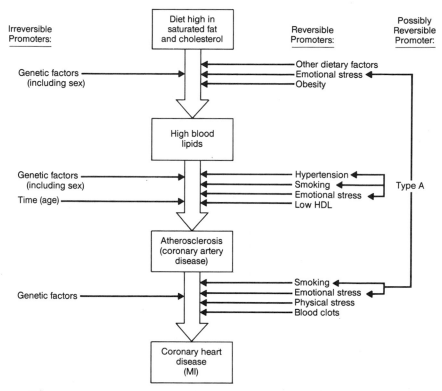

Figure 3.1 Chain of Causation: The Diet–Heart Hypothesis. (*Source:* Sherwin, R. (1978). Controlled trials of the diet-heart hypothesis: Some comments on the experimental unit. *American Journal of Epidemiology,* *108*, pp. 92–99.)

causation means that the element at the source of the arrow is, to some degree, a cause of the element at the point of the arrow.

In Figure 3.2 it can be seen that injection of hepatitis virus is one of the direct causes of jaundice in syphilis patients. This comes about through the injection of foreign (that is, from another person) serum, the presence of epidemic hepatitis in the community, and the biological characteristics of the hepatitis virus that allow it to survive and be transmitted in this fashion. The injection of foreign serum occurs due to intravenous injection as a treatment choice for syphilis, prior use of the same syringe for intravenous injection, serum remaining in the syringe from that use, and poor syringe hygiene that fails to eliminate the contamination.

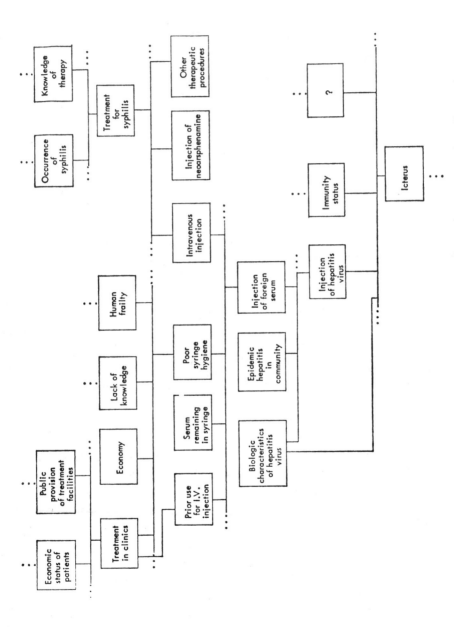

Figure 3.2 A Web of Causation for the Association Between Jaundice and Treatment for Syphilis. (*Source*: MacMahon, B., Pugh, T.F., & Ipsen, J. (1960). *Epidemiologic methods*. Boston: Little, Brown. p. 19.)

A later and more sophisticated, but rather generalized, web of causation was developed by Stallones (1966) to describe some of the interrelationships among the three major types of cardiovascular disease (see Figure 3.3). While this web does not attempt to provide a step-by-step description of the mechanisms by which the causal factors operate, it does give a clear view of how different factors may work together to produce one form or another of cardiovascular disease.

From the web of causation shown in Figure 3.3 we can see, for example, that hereditary tendencies, stress, and lack of physical activity contribute to hypertension (high blood pressure). This is also probably enhanced by atherosclerosis—the buildup of plaque on the inside walls of the arteries. Salt or sodium in the diet is also shown as possibly playing a role in causing hypertension, although the evidence for this factor is far less certain than the public and most health

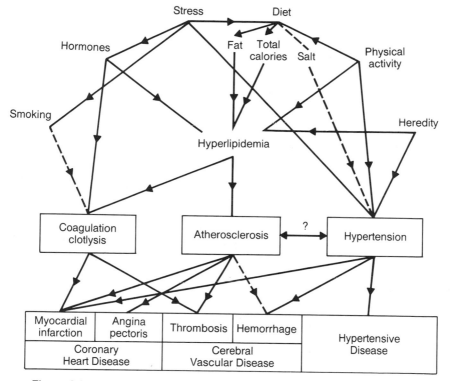

Figure 3.3 Web of Causation for the Major Cardiovascular Diseases. (*Source:* Stallones, R. A. (1966). Prospective epidemiologic studies of cerebrovascular disease. *Public Health Monograph No. 76*, Washington, DC: U.S. Government Printing Office. p. 53.)

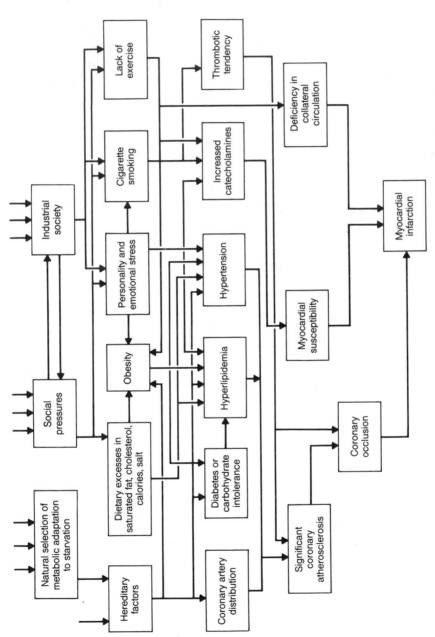

Figure 3.4   A Web of Causation for Myocardial Infarction. (*Source:* Friedman, G. D. (1980) *Primer of epidemiology.* New York: McGraw-Hill p. 4. Reprinted with permission.)

professionals seem to believe. Hypertension, then, in combination with atherosclerosis and the breakdown (lysis) of blood clots (resulting in a free-floating clot within the blood supply—an embolus) may cause a myocardial infarction (heart attack) when the clot lodges in one of the arteries constricted by atherosclerosis and blocks the blood flow to part of the heart muscle.

A more detailed web of causation for myocardial infarction (the classic "heart attack") developed by Friedman (1980) is shown in Figure 3.4. Complex though this web may seem, it is really only a beginning at mapping what is known about the etiology of heart disease.

A web of causation can be of great value in identifying possible points for preventive interventions. By examining Friedman's web of causation for myocardial infarction, for instance, we recognize that little can be done about the immediate causes of coronary occlusion (the artery is blocked by an embolus), atherosclerosis, myocardial susceptibility, or a deficiency of collateral circulation. By looking at the next level above this, however, we find hypertension, which is a possible point for intervention. We can treat hypertension with an array of highly effective drugs. A low-fat diet should, in most cases, help to reduce hyperlipidemia (excessive fats in the blood); we also have a growing ability to treat this condition with drugs. With these two interventions the risk of significant coronary atherosclerosis would be greatly reduced and that, in turn, would reduce the risk of heart disease.

Recommended Reading

MacMahon, B. Pugh, T. F., & Ipsen, J. (1960). *Epidemiologic methods.* Boston: Little, Brown.

Rothman, K. J. (1976). Causes. *American Journal of Epidemiology, 104,* 587–592.

Rothman, K. J., Greenland, S., & Walker, A. M. (1980). Concepts of interaction. *American Journal of Epidemiology, 112,* 465–466.

Susser, M. (1973). *Causal thinking in the health sciences: Concepts and strategies of epidemiology.* New York: Oxford University Press.

CHAPTER 4

The Natural History of Disease and the Spectrum of Health Services

There is a tendency to think of disease as an either–or proposition, like a light bulb that either is lit or is not. We think of ourselves as being either sick or well in almost equally simplistic terms.

A better analogy than the light bulb is the sunset—beginning as a faint glow in the eastern sky and gradually developing into full day-light; then, in the evening, gradually fading into the sunset. Similarly, disease develops gradually, not by distinct steps, but through a series of stages that merge into one another. This analogy breaks down when one considers that the development of disease lacks the certainty of the sunrise. Disease may develop slowly in one case and rapidly in another; it may fully develop in one case but fail to develop in another.

Time–Intensity Gradient of Disease

One way to describe the either–or process is by the time–intensity gradient described by Donabedian (1973). The concept of the time–intensity gradient is that disease develops first as small alterations in the microscopic structure or functioning of a few cells of the host body. As the disease process continues, its impact on the host increases, in terms of both the number of cells affected and the extent of the alterations. At first the alterations are imperceptible to the host but as their impact increases the host begins to experience symptoms of the disease. Eventually, if the alterations continue to increase in their

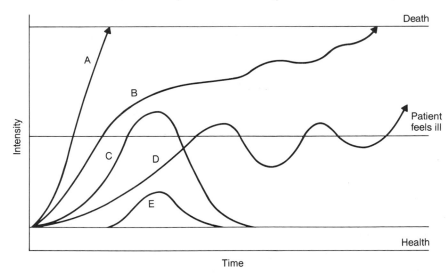

Figure 4.1   Some Hypothetical Time–Intensity Relationships in Disease. (*Source:* Donabedian, A. (1973). *Aspects of medical care administration: Specifying requirements for health care.* Cambridge, MA: Harvard University Press, Commonwealth Fund.)

intensity, the host identifies the symptoms as constituting an illness and may seek treatment.

The disease process may follow a range of different courses. It may proceed rapidly or slowly. It may continue to increase in intensity until it results in death of the host or it may reach some peak and then wane as the host recovers fully or partially. It may never reach a sufficient degree of intensity for the host to become aware of it at all. With some diseases, such as multiple sclerosis or relapsing fever, the course of the disease may be one of sporadic attacks with symptom-free periods in between. There is one such course for each disease that is the usual course for the untreated disease—it may be called its *natural history*. These alternative courses are illustrated in Figure 4.1.

A Continuum of Health Status

We may describe the vertical axis of the time-intensity gradient as being divisible into the stages of subclinical disease and clinical disease. Although the absence of disease is often treated as a single stage called health, it may be usefully divided into two or more stages.

We will conceptualize it as containing the stages of high-level wellness and of susceptibility, which will provide us with a simple continuum of health status or a wellness–illness continuum.

Stages of High-Level Wellness

The concept of high-level wellness, or simply wellness, was introduced by Holbert L. Dunn, first Director of the National Center for Health Statistics, to describe a stage of health that was beyond the mere absence of disease or susceptibility. Dunn (1961) defines high-level wellness as, "an integrated method of functioning which is oriented toward maximizing the potential of which the individual is capable" (p. 4). Dunn's definition is similar to Maslow's (1956) psychological concept of self-actualization.

Wellness is not a negative condition, definable by what the person is not (sick or susceptible) or by what the person does not have or do (risk factors). It is a positive, dynamic condition of interaction with the environment, which is optimal for growth. Ardell (1982) uses simpler words than Dunn but says essentially the same thing when he defines wellness as "a lifestyle approach for realizing your best possibilities for well-being" (p. 14). Wellness is not focused on avoiding illness, Ardell emphasizes, but rather, it "is targeted to the enjoyable, lifelong quest for attainable peaks of optimal whole-person functioning as its own reward" (p. 21).

John Travis (Ryan & Travis, 1981) describes an illness–wellness continuum in which the wellness arm of his continuum is divisible into stages of education, growth, and self-actualization. Ardell (1982), on the other hand, divides this end of the continuum into two stages: intermediate-level tinkering with health and high-level wellness. The intermediate level is characterized by "sporadic efforts toward better health," while high-level wellness is an integrated state of "whole person excellence" (p. 20). Such further subdivision of the stage of wellness is probably a good idea, although at present there is little empirical basis for identifying stages of wellness that lead to high-level wellness. Until more evidence is accumulated, some may choose to accept Travis' or Ardell's version, while others may prefer to wait until more evidence is available before thinking of the stages of wellness.

Neutral Point

Travis' (Ryan and Travis, 1981) illness–wellness continuum is a double-headed arrow centered on a "neutral point" at which there is no discernible illness and no discernible wellness. In terms of the continuum described here, we would place this point between the stage of susceptibility and the stage of wellness. Travis makes the point that traditional medicine can only bring one to the neutral point; it does not address the wellness side of the continuum at all. Similarly, epidemiology has traditionally only looked at the illness side of the continuum of health status. The epidemiologic examination of positive health states is only in its infancy.

Stage of Susceptibility

During the stage of susceptibility, the disease process is not present but factors that favor its occurrence are present. For instance, cigarette smoking, high blood pressure, and elevated serum cholesterol can set the groundwork for ischemic heart disease. Factors such as these, whose presence are associated with an increased probability that disease will develop later, are called *risk factors*. The presence of risk factors means that the occurrence of the disease is more likely—it does not guarantee that the disease will occur.

Stage of Subclinical Disease

During the stage of subclinical disease, the host is not aware of an ongoing disease process. The intensity of the changes wrought in the host's body is not yet great enough to be experienced as symptoms. Because the host does not experience symptoms and thus has no awareness of the disease, medical attention is not sought. If the disease process is discovered in the course of a periodic physical examination or a screening program, it may be more treatable at this time than after it has reached the stage of clinical disease—this is not always so, but often it is.

If the intensity continues to increase, then the stage of clinical illness will be reached. In many instances, however, the intensity does not continue to increase and the disease process eventually fades away without ever being recognized by the host. Such instances are known as *abortive cases*.

Stage of Clinical Disease

During the stage of clinical disease, the host becomes aware of the alterations in functioning or structure that result from the disease process. The alterations may now be referred to as symptoms of disease. As the host's awareness of the symptoms increases, the host may either engage in denial (refusing to admit that the symptoms do represent underlying disease) or adopt some variety of sick role behavior. This sick role behavior may involve efforts at self-care, seeking care or advice from nonprofessionals, or seeking medical care.

If the stage of clinical illness persists for a long period of time (commonly thought of as 60 days or longer), the disease might be said to have passed into a stage of chronicity. Alternatively, death and long-term disability might also be seen as stages beyond the clinical disease stage. Fortunately, in most cases the stage after clinical illness is a return to the subclinical stage and via that to some improved level of health.

Levels of Prevention _____

The literature on public health has long described the prevention of disease in terms of three levels. *Primary prevention* is the reduction of incidence by lowering the number of new cases of disease occurring. *Secondary prevention* is the reduction of prevalence through the early detection and cure of disease, because this may reduce the transmission of disease from host to host and may also reduce the incidence of disease. *Tertiary prevention* is the prevention of long-term disability or death due to a disease.

Primary Prevention

Primary prevention activities take place during the stage of susceptibility. They include such strategies as eliminating risk factors from the environment, erecting barriers between risk factors and potential hosts, changing the behavior of potential hosts so as to reduce exposure to risk factors, decreasing the effect of risk factors on potential hosts, or making potential hosts stronger and more resistant to disease.

The elimination of risk factors from the environment and the erection of barriers between risk factors and potential hosts are traditional public health activities. Attempts to control air and water pollution, for instance, fall into this category. Sewage disposal systems and auto seat belts can both be seen as examples of erecting barriers between people and the forces that might cause us harm.

Changing host behavior is one of the most important strategies for primary prevention of the major threats to life and health in contemporary society. Former Surgeon General Julius Richmond in *Healthy People* (1979) states that

> Within the grasp of most Americans are simple measures to enhance the prospects of good health, including: elimination of cigarette smoking; reduction of alcohol misuse; moderate dietary changes to reduce intake of excess calories, fat, salt and sugar; moderate exercise; periodic screening... for major disorders such as high blood pressure and certain cancers; and adherence to speed laws and use of seat belts. (p. 10)

Vaccination is the most obvious example of prevention by decreasing the effect of agents on potential hosts. Stress management programs, which teach progressive relaxation or meditation, are prevention efforts that attempt to lessen the impact of stress on the individual.

Secondary Prevention

Secondary prevention efforts take place during the stage of subclinical disease. Its approach to prevention attempts to get diseased individuals into treatment as early as possible. It is generally assumed that earlier intervention will result in a shorter duration of the disease and lessened chance of severe illness or death. However, its assumption is not always valid. In some diseases earlier detection only means a longer period of treatment without shortening the course of the disease or reducing its severity. Thus, secondary prevention is not an appropriate strategy for all diseases.

Secondary prevention is often carried out by mass screening. A relatively simple test is applied to a large apparently healthy population. The results of the test divide the population into those who probably have the disease and those who probably do not. Persons in the former group are referred to a physician for diagnosis to determine whether they, in fact, do have the disease.

An alternate approach to secondary prevention is the education of the public to recognize early signs of disease that might otherwise be overlooked. The American Cancer Society's efforts to familiarize all Americans with the seven warning signs of cancer is one example of the approach to secondary prevention. Breast self-examination for women and testicular self-examination for men are also instances of its approach.

Tertiary Prevention

Tertiary prevention takes place during the stage of clinical disease and may extend into the stage of disability. Tertiary prevention tries to keep illness from resulting in long-term after-effects for the host—it represents a focus on reducing the virulence of the disease.

Much of the efforts of tertiary prevention take place in the stage of disability and are concerned with the limitation of disability and rehabilitation. Limitation of disability refers to efforts to minimize the after-effects of disease—restoring motion and preventing contractures in a damaged limb, for instance. The term rehabilitation literally means to restore to a former way of living. It is an attempt to restore the disabled individual to a productive and hopefully self-sufficient role in society.

A Spectrum of Health Services

A somewhat broader framework for describing the full range of health services has been proposed by some public health workers. The framework describes health services as divisible into areas of health promotion, health maintenance, and health restoration (see Figure 4.2). The same concepts are found in *Healthy People: The Surgeon General's Report on Health Promotion and Disease Prevention* (1979, p. 119) but here they are called health promotion, disease prevention, and medical care.

Health Promotion

Health promotion refers to measures targeted at healthy (disease-free) individuals with the aim of further improving their level of health. The goal of these measures is the attainment of high-level wellness.

Health promotion has often been used as a synonym for primary prevention or even as a subdivision of primary prevention. It seems, however, to be a term with a meaning well worth preserving in its own right. With the increasing public and professional interest in the wellness concept, health promotion in its proper sense is likely to receive increasing usage.

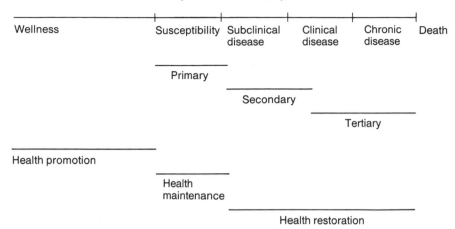

Figure 4.2 Health Services and Health Status.

Health Maintenance

Health maintenance refers to measures targeted at healthy (disease-free) individuals with the aim of preventing the development of disease. This level of health services is identical with primary prevention.

The use of the term *health maintenance organization (HMO)* for prepaid medical care arrangements (which we would call health restoration) causes some confusion. This term was apparently chosen for such plans because of the incentive in a prepayment plan for physicians to practice preventive medicine. In other words, if the HMO can practice primary prevention on its members, it will need to provide less of more expensive medical care, and because the prepayment remains the same it will thus make a bigger profit. In an HMO, the profit motive was to encourage efforts at health maintenance rather than health restoration. How well this works in practice is subject to dispute.

Health Restoration

Health restoration refers to measures targeted at sick individuals with the aim of restoring them to their previous disease-free state. This incorporates the whole range of what is commonly called medical care. The alternate term, however, recognizes that health restoration is not the domain of physicians alone. Not only do other health-care providers (such as nurses, podiatrists, and optometrists) play important roles in health restoration, but so do nonprofessional caregivers (such as parents and spouses), and so does self-care.

Recommended Readings

Duncan, D. F., & Gold, R. S. (1986). Reflections: Health promotion—what is it? *Health Values, 10*(3), 47–48.

Ibrahim, M.A. (1983). Epidemiology: Application to health services. *Journal of Health Administration Education, 1*(1), 37–69.

Regier, D. A., Goldberg, I. D., & Taube, C. A. (1978). The de facto U.S. mental health services system. *Archives of General Psychiatry, 35,* 685–693.

PART II

The Vital Statistics

It is now difficult to realize how little was known about the health of the nation or about the health of any of its political subdivisions as recently as 50 years ago. At that time, there were only four general sources of information: death statistics, reports of notifiable diseases, prevalence of illness from two U.S. Censuses, and a few scattered surveys of illness prevalence and incidence. Each of these sources provided data that was unsatisfactory on several counts.

— *G. Comstock (1974, p. ii)*

Today we have a vast array of sources of data on the public's health, as will be seen in Chapter 5. Chapter 6 presents the various measures used with data on births and deaths, while Chapter 7 reviews the principal measures of disease and disability. These measures, for the most part, take the form of rates or ratios.

A proportion expresses the comparative relation between a part of a thing and the whole. It is usually expressed as a percentage. An example would be that in the 1980 Census 13.1 percent of the U.S. population was aged 65 or older.

A rate is a type of proportion that reflects the probability of occurrence of some particular event in a defined population at risk. A rate takes this form:

$$\frac{x}{y} \times k$$

where

x = Number of times an event has occurred during a specified interval of time.

y = Number of persons who were at risk of the event occurring to them.

$k =$ A constant—any round number large enough that
multiplying it times the dividend of x divided
by y will result in a number greater than one.

A ratio expresses the relationship between two quantities, x and y, in which all the events in quantity x did not necessarily occur to the persons in quantity y. A ratio takes this form:

$$x:y \quad \text{or} \quad \frac{x}{y} \times k$$

Numerous examples will be found in the chapters that follow.

CHAPTER 5

Sources of Information About Health

Robert S. Gold, Ph.D., Dr.P.H.
Project Director, 1990 Objectives Initiative
Office of Disease Prevention and Health Promotion
Department of Health and Human Services

Charles E. Basch, Ph.D.
Assistant Professor
Teacher's College—Columbia University

Types of Health-Related Data _____

When we think about data related to health, we most often think about morbidity (illness) and mortality (death) statistics. However, as we will see, morbidity and mortality statistics are only part of the vast array of data that we can use in health education. There are, in fact, five major sources of population data that are of some value to health educators. These five include the following:

1. Demographic information about populations. The term *demography* generally refers to the study of human populations, and demographers are interested in data regarding the makeup and distribution of these populations. Demographic information is collected in a variety of ways, including regular and special censuses, and by gathering vital statistics data.

Among the most important tasks of demographers are the following:

1. To ascertain the number, characteristics, and distribution of people in a given area.
2. To determine what and how changes are occurring in the population.
3. To estimate, on this basis, future trends.

In order to accomplish these principal goals, demographers use simple tools, such as counting for data collection; rates, ratios, proportions, and indices for data analysis; and mathematical models for prediction.

It is possible to describe demography as having two separate elements—a static component and a dynamic component. The static component, sometimes called descriptive demography, focuses on the description of the size, composition, and distribution of human populations. Here the demographer is interested in information regarding the number of individuals within a given population, their specific characteristics (e.g., age distribution, racial composition, marital status, and so forth), and how the population is distributed in a given geographic area. Such information is generally collected in censuses and special surveys.

The dynamic component of demography is concerned with how population changes over time. There are three principal factors affecting population change—births, deaths, and migration (both in-migration and out-migration). Birth and death records are generally compiled as part of a vital statistics system. In this country, all 50 states are part of a national registry of births and deaths. We do not, however, have a good source of reliable information regarding migration in human populations. The balancing equation that follows illustrates the relationship between each of these components and population changes:

$$PT = P + B - D + I - O + e$$

where

PT = total population at a given time.

P = initial population.

B = number of births during a given period of time.

D = number of deaths during a given period of time.

I = in-migration during a given period of time.

O = out-migration during a given period of time.

e = error in measurement.

This formula, referred to as *decomposition of population change,* illustrates the general relationship between the factors that affect population change over time. It is not, however, a precise model for predicting population change.

Sources of Demographic Information

There are three principal sources of information that demographers use regularly: censuses, special surveys, and registration systems. The latter two will be discussed later in this chapter in the broader context of health surveys and vital statistics systems.

Censuses. A census is a means of compiling descriptive information on human populations. The term *census* refers to data collection on the entire population rather than on a sample of the population. The variety of U.S. census data is shown in Exhibit 5.1.

The United Nations recommends that censuses maintain the following characteristics for the greatest return:

1. There should be individual enumeration, that is, the unit of counting should be the individual. When the census was first done in the United States, the unit of counting was the family, not the individual. It was not until our sixth census, the census of 1850, that the unit of enumeration was the individual.

2. There should be universality within defined territories. This is another way of saying that each individual should be counted, regardless of his or her personal, professional, or social characteristics. Again, our early censuses in this country considered only whites; blacks were excluded.

3. There should be simultaneity, that is, the entire census should be concluded on a single day. In a practical sense, this is not possible for large censuses. However, the intent is valid, and data collection for censuses should be concluded in as short a period as possible. The principal reason for this is the dynamic nature of human populations; they are changing constantly. If census taking were stretched out over a long period of time, data collected initially would no longer be as precise as data collected at a later time.

4. There should be defined periodicity, that is, census taking should be done on a regular basis. In the United States, censuses were typically conducted on a decennial basis—every 10 years. However, currently there are plans for 5-year censuses to be

EXHIBIT 5.1   General Census Publications

A. Population And Housing Census Reports

   1. PHC80–1 Block Statistics
   2. PCH80–2 Census Tracts
   3. PCH80–3 Summary Characteristics for Governmental Units and Standard Metropolitan Statistical Areas
   4. PCH80–4 Congressional Districts of the 89th Congress
   5. PCH80–S1–1 Provisional Estimates of Social, Economic, and Housing Characteristics
   6. PCH80–S2 Advance Estimates of Social, Economic, and Housing Characteristics

B. Population Census Reports

   1. PC80–1 Volume 1: Characteristics of the Population
   2. PC80–1–A Chapter A: Number of Inhabitants
   3. PC80–1–B Chapter B: General Population Characteristics
   4. PC80–1–C Chapter C: General Social and Economic Characteristics
   5. PC80–1–D Chapter D: Detailed Population Characteristics
   6. PC80–2 Volume 2: Subject Reports
   7. PC80–S1 Supplementary Reports

C. Housing Census Reports

   1. HC80–1 Volume 1: Characteristics of Housing Units
   2. HC80–1–A Chapter A: General Housing Characteristics
   3. HC80–1–B Chapter B: Detailed Housing Characteristics
   4. HC80–2 Volume 2: Metropolitan Housing Characteristics
   5. HC80–3 Volume 3: Subject Reports
   6. HC80–4 Volume 4: Components of Inventory Change
   7. HC80–5 Volume 5: Residential Finance
   8. HC80–S1–1: Supplementary Reports

D. Evaluation and Reference Reports

   1. PCH80–E Evaluation and Research Reports
   2. PCH80–R Reference Reports
   PCH80–R1: User's Guide
   PCH80–R2: History
   PCH80–R3: Alphabetical Index of Industries and Occupations
   PCH80–R4: Classified Index of Industries and Occupations
   PCH80–R5: Geographic Identification Code Scheme

conducted. Since population changes so rapidly in the United States, a 10-year census loses its utility in a very short period of time. Therefore, we will move to a 5-year census to update our data more frequently.

5. There should be sponsorship by a national government. This is recommended to assure continuity and regularity, as well as to assure that the principal aims of regular census taking are not replaced with the aims of current power groups or lobbies.

2. Social and business statistics may also be of some use to us in health education. Examples of some useful social and business statistics include the gross national product (GNP), employment rates, welfare status, and inflation rates. These are most often tabulated at national and state levels; however, there are other statistics that are often collected locally as well. Examples of such statistics include daily school attendance records and local manufacturing and industrial data. It is worth examining some examples of how such statistics may be useful to health educators.

Health care expenditures as a percentage of the GNP give us some evidence of the magnitude of growth in the health-care system over time and how it is relative to the growth of our economy. The fact that this proportion has been rising dramatically in the last decade has been alarming to many in the health-care field as well as to consumers.

3. Records detailing social and political events of significance to the population. Such records include the voting records of elected representatives on specific health issues, or information on municipal and metropolitan areas and national governmental institutions and events. As health educators become more politically astute, they will begin to monitor voting records of local, state, and national representatives, on issues particularly related to health. These voting records may then be used to help decide which politicians to support.

4. Data on health resources, such as counts of the numbers of health professionals and students in professional training programs. Such resources also include in-patient, out-patient, ancillary health, and related facilities.

5. Data on the number of persons suffering from illness and disability or residing in health-care institutions (morbidity data), and the number of persons who have died (mortality data).

Although all of these types of data may be of some value to professionals working in health-related fields, it is important to note that all of the information is not equally reliable. Some attention must be paid to the originating source of the information, the procedures followed in assembling and aggregating the information, and matters of the precision and reliability of the information.

Health Information Resources _____

Although each of these sources of data has its appropriate applications to the health sciences, Pearce (1985) notes that in order to provide an appropriate overview of the broad scope of resources, we should use several criteria to narrow the field. Following on her lead, we will only review sources that have the following characteristics:

Selection Characteristics
1. They are national in coverage or representative of the situation in the country as a whole.
2. They are currently operational, although they may be periodic in their collection of data.
3. They must be operated by either the federal government or the private sector.
4. They must produce primary data rather than a secondary compilation of data from other sources.

Pearce (1985) states also that the application of such criteria excludes state level sources, which can be valuable for some applications, and several compendia that contain data extracted from primary data sources. Examples of these compendia include the *Statistical Abstract of the United States*, compiled by the Bureau of the Census; *Health— United States*, the annual report of the Secretary of the Department of Health and Human Services; and *Prevention*, a biannual publication of the Office of Disease Prevention and Health Promotion, Department of Health and Human Services.

Pearce (1985) then provides a framework for the organization of such diverse sets of information. She proposes three broad groupings:

1. Health status indicators, including morbidity and mortality;
2. Health care resources and their utilization;
3. Health economics.

You can see from Pearce's list that it is slightly narrower in scope than our original listing of potential data sources. This should not, however, suggest that the other sources are less important, as Rice (1985) points out:

> [I]t is important to understand that state and local agencies have key interests and roles in the collection and use of health statistics, including

state and local health agencies, health planning agencies, rate review bodies, mental health agencies, Governors' offices, legislators, and universities. Many of these data systems have been developed with funding assistance from the Federal government either directly or indirectly through service delivery grants.

The recent shift from categorical health programs to block grants, the cutbacks in federal funding, and the lack of federal requirements for accountability will adversely affect our ability to adequately track and monitor the impact of these programs on the health of the poor, children and mothers, and the elderly, as well as on institutions serving the poor. (p. 19)

Caveats in Selecting Sources

Although we will review several strengths and weaknesses of each of the data bases, you should recognize that there are some general issues that are cross-cutting. These issues deserve special attention in attempting to evaluate the usefulness of a specific data source.

1. Population based surveys obtain socioeconomic data, family characteristics, and information on the impact of illness, such as days lost from work or limitation of activity. These data are limited by the amount of information a respondent remembers or is willing to impart.
2. Detailed medical information, such as precise diagnoses or the types of operations performed, may not be known and so will not be reported.
   Conversely, health care providers, such as physicians and hospitals, usually have good diagnostic information but little or no information about the socioeconomic characteristics of the individuals or the impact of illnesses on individuals.
3. The population covered by different data collection systems may not be the same, and understanding the differences is critical to interpreting the data.
4. Data on vital statistics and national expenditures cover the entire population. Most data on morbidity and utilization of health resources cover only the civilian noninstitutionalized population. Thus, statistics are not included for military personnel, who are usually young; for institutionalized people, who may be any age; or for nursing home residents, who are usually old.
5. All data collection systems are subject to error, and records may be incomplete or contain inaccurate information. People may not remember essential information, a question may not mean the same thing to different respondents, and some institutions or individuals may not respond at all. It is not always possible to measure the magnitude of these errors.
6. Overall estimates generally have relatively small sampling errors, but estimates for certain population subgroups may be based on small numbers and have relatively large sampling errors.

7. Some data on natality is based on sampling strategies and some on enumeration of the entire population. Where the data are based on complete counts there is no sampling error. However, you should recognize that where the actual number of events is small, considerable caution should be exercised in interpreting these data. When there are small counts, these numbers are subject to extreme variability based on random fluctuations and are considered generally unreliable. (National Center for Health Statistics, 1985, p. 158)

To these caveats, Rice (1985) adds the following:

8. There are many attempts at standardization of data elements in national studies, the use of uniform definitions and coding, and agreement on minimum data sets for studies. Such standardization leads to our ability to compare and aggregate data across studies. Examples of such efforts include standard classification schemes for race and ethnicity implemented by all Federal agencies in their data collection activities as a result of standards set by the Office of Management and Budget. There has been some Federal movement toward minimum data sets under the auspices of the National Committee on Vital and Health Statistics; and the International Classification of Diseases, 9th Revision (Clinical Modification) is now widely used for coding medical conditions and hospital discharge data. However, "the coding of surgical procedures, ambulatory care visits, and drugs... have not been standardized."
9. There are many issues of confidentiality, freedom of information, and invasion of privacy and their impact on data collection. There exists a conflict between a public's right to know, and an individual's right to privacy. (p. 19)

Sources of Data

It is time now to look specifically at several sources of health data. We will utilize Pearce's (1985) framework to structure this section of the chapter. You should keep in mind the caveats reviewed in the previous section. In each case, several examples will be cited; however, there will be an extended discussion of only one or two of the sources from each of three categories.

Health Status Data

National Vital Statistics System. Through this system, the National Center for Health Statistics (NCHS) collects and publishes data on births, deaths, marriages, and divorces in the United States. Fetal deaths are classified and tabulated separately from other deaths. It should be noted that registration of basic vital statistics is the responsibility of local areas and states, but, with the use of uniform registration practices and cooperative agreements between jurisdictions, the NCHS is able to collect, aggregate, and publish summary statistics in these areas. NCHS collects data from all states, New York City, the District of Columbia, Puerto Rico, the U.S. Virgin Islands, and Guam.

Provisional data are tabulated and published monthly (*Monthly Vital Statistics Report*), and there is also an annual summary. Provisional death rates categorized by case, age, race, and sex are estimated from the current mortality sample—a 10 percent sample of death certificates from all participating jurisdictions.

Uses of Vital Statistics. Vital statistics data provide us with our best estimates of births, deaths, marriages, and divorces. Anyone interested in tabulating the leading causes of death for a given population, or death and birth rates by age, sex, and race will find these data useful. "Followback" surveys indicate that the coverage is extensive, with more than 99 percent of all births accounted for. Although no similar estimates are available for deaths, it is believed that these data are just as complete.

Caveats. On-going registration systems are typically maintained to record and monitor vital events, such as live births, still births, deaths, marriages, and divorces. The following characteristics are considered minimal for an adequate registration system to operate.

1. A registration system is best operated by a national government or some executive agency of a national government. In the U.S., the NCHS collects and tabulates vital statistics data but local and state collection of the original data is also a part of the system.
2. In order to provide adequate data, there should be uniform records used for vital events. Although uniform records are recommended in the U.S., each jurisdiction makes some variation to suit local needs.
3. Universality within defined territories should be provided. (Geographic coverage for births and deaths in the U.S. has been complete since 1933.)
4. A specified maximum interval between the occurrence of an event and its recording in the system are necessary. Although records are supposed to be transmitted to NCHS at specified intervals, we still depend on the local areas to comply with this. They are not

always able to do so and the current mortality sample contains a sampling of death data based on a sample of records collected each month—regardless of when the event occurred.

A related problem is that final data publications run several years behind. In 1986, the 1980 data are available in final publication.

5. Data should be tabulated based on date of occurrence; *not* based on date of report or recording. This is preferred, although not always possible.
6. Place of residence (de jure) is a more useful tabulation technique than is place of occurrence (de facto).

Vital registration systems should be designed to make the information accessible, to provide for complete and useable information, and to enable the information to be processed for statistical purposes.

Health and Nutrition Examination Survey. An excellent example of the kind of data collected related to health status is the *National Health and Nutrition Examination Survey (NHANES)*. This survey was initiated in the National Center for Health Statistics (NCHS) in 1970 and the first phase of NHANES was conducted from 1971–1974. NHANES I was an extension and modification of another regular survey conducted by NCHS a decade earlier—the Health Examination Survey (HES). NHANES differs from HES by the addition of a new area of responsibility to the National Center's data collection efforts—measurement of nutritional status of the population and surveillance of that status over time. To accomplish this objective, data were collected on the nutritional status of American people through dietary intake data, biochemical tests, physical measurements, and clinical assessments for evidence of nutritional deficiency. Detailed examinations were given to some by dentists, ophthalmologists, and dermatologists. In addition, data were collected from a sample of adults on overall health care needs and behavior, and more detailed examination data were collected on cardiovascular, respiratory, arthritic, and hearing conditions.

NHANES I's target population was the civilian noninstitutionalized population 1–74 years of age in the United States, excluding those living on reservation lands. The study involved household interviews of 28,043 persons, with a 70 percent (20,749) completion rate. A subsample of persons aged 25–74 years was selected to receive a more detailed health examination and groups at high risk of malnutrition were oversampled.

A second round for NHANES (NHANES II) was conducted in the civilian noninstitutionalized population 6 months to 74 years of age residing in the United States. This round was conducted between 1976 and 1980. Although the nutritional component remained comparable to NHANES I, emphasis on the medical area was shifted to diabetes, kidney and liver functions, allergy, and speech pathology. NHANES II has a sample of 27,801 persons, with a 73 percent completion rate (20,322).

Uses. The data available from NHANES rounds I and II are extensive. These data will be useful whenever a researcher wants national probability data related to nutritional status, health status in general, and health behaviors. The maintenance of a standard set of items through the first two rounds provides the capacity for longitudinal data—although not panel data. These data are useful also for comparing local and regional data to national data.

Caveats. Although extensive in coverage, the general caveats related to coding and tabulating errors are most important. Problems may exist with some dietary data—particularly that related to fiber in the earlier round—because the definition of dietary fiber may change over time.

Other Examples of Health Status Data.

1. National morbidity and mortality reporting systems, maintained by the Centers for Disease Control. This is a weekly publication of current data on notifiable diseases and related data (*Morbidity and Mortality Weekly Report*).
2. *Drug Abuse Warning Network* operated by the National Institute on Drug Abuse. This report monitors trends in illicit drug use.
3. *National Health Interview Survey,* conducted by the National Center for Health Statistics. This is the major source of information on the health of Americans. Conducted annually since 1957, it is a nationwide sample survey of households on demographic characteristics, illnesses, injuries, impairments, chronic conditions, utilization of health resources, and other topics.
4. *U.S. Immunization Survey.* This is the result of a cooperative effort between the Centers for Disease Control and the U.S. Bureau of the Census. Estimates are based on data collected from a subsample of households interviewed for the Current Population Survey or the Bureau of the Census.

Resource Utilization

National Master Facility Inventory. This inventory is compiled by the National Center for Health Statistics and is a comprehensive file of in-patient health facilities in the U.S. Included in this inventory are three categories of facilities: hospitals, nursing and related care homes, and other custodial care facilities. More than 33,000 facilities are represented in this survey conducted between 1968 and 1975. Since 1976, all the data have been collected by the American Hospital Association.

Included in this survey is information about the types of facilities, services offered, size, in-patient days of care, ownership, discharge, procedures, fiscal matters, and staffing.

Uses. Such data as these can be very useful in examining the relationship between facility type and operations, and outcomes. In addition, it is possible to track facility growth over time and to compare local resources with those on a regional or national level. The data are useful also for producing statistics on each of the facility types.

Caveats. These data are provided by the facilities themselves. Under-reporting and overreporting are possible. In addition, the updating of the inventory will be behind actual data.

Other Examples of Sources on Resource Utilization.

1. *National Hospital Discharge Survey.* Conducted by the National Center for Health Statistics. This is the principal source of information on in-patient utilization of short-stay hospitals.
2. *National Nursing Home Survey.* The National Center for Health Statistics conducted two sample surveys (1974 and 1977) on nursing homes to collect information on expenditures, residents, staff, and discharged patients.
3. *National Ambulatory Medical Care Survey.* This is a continuing survey of ambulatory medical encounters conducted by the National Center for Health Statistics.
4. *Surveys of Mental Health Facilities.* Conducted by the National Institute of Mental Health, the Survey and Reports Branch of the Division of Biometry and Epidemiology.

Health Economics

National Medical Care Expenditure Survey (NMCES). Conducted by the National Center for Health Statistics, NMCES provides detailed national estimates on the utilization and expenditures for various types of medical care. The first wave of this survey was conducted in 1980 and provided data on a national sample of civilian noninstitutionalized Americans, as well as a separate survey of those eligible for Medicaid in several states. A third survey of administrative records was designed to verify data collected from the other surveys. Each respondent was interviewed three times beginning in February 1980 and running through March 1981. A second round is now in the final planning stages.

Uses. For those who need detailed expenditure data on health resources, the NMCES is an indispensible source of information. Included in the data are health insurance coverage, episodes of illness, hospital admissions, bed days, restricted activity days, physician and dental visits, other medical encounters, and purchases of prescribed medications.

Caveats. As with other data related to self-reports, these data depend on respondents' abilities to recall and their interest in honest reporting. However, the verification provided by the administrative records audit provides powerful support to the utility of the data.

Consumer Price Index (CPI). The CPI is a monthly measure of price change for a fixed "market basket" of goods and services. Revised periodically, it provides an estimate of the way in which Americans buy products and services. The CPI is available from the Bureau of Labor Statistics, Department of Labor.

In this chapter we reviewed a select number of sources of information but you should recognize that much more exists than we are able to describe here. More extensive listings can be found in NCHS (1985), and Mullner, Byre, and Killingsworth (1983).

Summary

Review of data sources for health information can be extensive, including the results of published research and other publications such as books, newspapers, and voting records of politicians. At the national level there are many data systems that have been established to document the health status of population subgroups and that can provide data useful to local and regional needs. The Vital Registration system, with its data on natality, deaths, marriages and divorces; the national morbidity and mortality reporting system, with its data on reportable diseases; and the National Hospital Discharge Survey are several examples.

Although we did not focus on local data in this chapter, it is also often available from health departments or local planning agencies. These data are also useful for estimating population risk and for calculating local rates. These rates may then be compared with national data to make decisions about resource allocation and program need at the local level. Statewide data can be useful in terms of sociodemographic composition of the population.

Although it should be evident that many sources of data exist, you should be cognizant of the potential problems with any data set. We have reviewed some of the major ones here. To summarize, you should remember that many potential problems exist. Among the most important are:

1. Sampling errors that can result in undercoverage or overestimation of population characteristics.
2. Respondent and investigator errors.
3. Errors resulting from nonresponse.
4. Editing and data processing errors.

With these caveats in mind, you should utilize data within the constraints of your knowledge or the reliability and validity of the data you are interested in.

Recommended Reading

National Vital Statistics System

National Center for Health Statistics. (1984). *Vital statistics of the United States, 1980*, Vol. I. DHHS Pub. No. (PHS) 85–1100; Vol. II, Part A. DHHS Pub. No. (PHS) 84–1101, Public Health Service. Washington, DC: U.S. Government Printing Office.

NHANES I

Miller, H. W. (February 1973). *Plan and operation of the National Health and Nutrition Examination Survey, United States, 1971–1973*. National Center for Health Statistics. Vital and Health Statistics, Series 1—Nos. 10a and 10b. DHEW Pub. No. (HSM) 73–1310, Health Services and Mental Health Administration. Washington, DC: U.S. Government Printing Office.

NHANES II

McDowell, A., Engel, A., Massey, J. T., & Maurer, K. (July 1981). *Plan and operation of the second National Health and Nutrition Examination Survey, 1976–1980.* National Center for Health Statistics. Vital and Health Statistics, Series 1–No. 15, DHHS Pub. No. (PHS) 81–1317, Public Health Service. Washington, DC: U.S. Government Printing Office.

National Master Facility Inventory

Hollis, G. G. (January 1971). *Design and methodology of the 1967 Master Facility Inventory Survey.* National Center for Health Statistics. Vital and Health Statistics, PHS Pub. No. 1000 Series 1—No. 9, Public Health Service. Washington, DC: U.S. Government Printing Office.

CHAPTER **6**

Measures of Natality and Mortality

①
Among the statistics of greatest epidemiologic importance are the traditional vital statistics—rates of births, deaths, marriages, and divorces. Because the calculations for marriage and divorce rates are relatively straightforward, and are not usually of epidemiologic interest, this chapter will examine only the rates of births and deaths.

Natality Measures

②
Natality rates measure additions or probable additions to a population—in other words, live births. Natality is most often measured in terms of period rates that describe the childbearing experience of a population on an annual, or other time period, basis. Natality may ③ also be expressed in terms of cohort rates, which describe the reproductive history of a select group of women up to a specified age.

The term *live birth* would seem to be self-explanatory but the operation of a statistical reporting system requires a relatively precise ④ definition of the events to be counted. A live birth is usually defined as any product of conception that shows any sign of life after complete birth. Such signs of life include heart beat, respiration, crying, pulsation of the umbilical cord, or movement of the voluntary muscles.
⑤
The crude birth rate relates live births to the total population (of both sexes and all ages) for a specific interval of time, usually one year.

$$\text{Crude birth rate} = \frac{\begin{array}{c}\text{Number of live births}\\ \text{during time interval}\end{array}}{\text{Total population}} \times 1{,}000$$

A serious methodological problem arises in calculating the crude birth rate or any other rate that is calculated for a period of time rather than cross-sectionally for one point in time. This problem involves the fact that most populations change over time. If the population was changing during the interval for which rate is calculated, what population figure is used as the denominator?

The best answer to this question is to use the average population for the interval. The average population for a year may be calculated easily by summing the population on January 1, the population on January 2, the population on January 3, and so on through December 31, then dividing this sum by 365 (or 366 for a leap year). The problem with this solution is not the simple though lengthy calculation, but the difficulty in obtaining daily population figures. The U.S. Census is taken once every 10 years, not daily. Daily population counts are available for jails, prisons, schools, hospitals, and military institutions, but not for cities, towns, states, or nations.

The solution to this problem found in almost every text is to use the midinterval population. Thus, for an annual crude birth rate, the population on July 1 of that year would be used as the denominator. This solution is offered as though it actually makes sense; as though a census was actually conducted each year on July 1 for the convenience of epidemiologists. In fact, we must settle for the best population statistic available, which more often than not is the last Census figure. This problem, and its lack of a satisfactory solution, applies as well to all of the period rates discussed in this text.

Another problem is that, because age and sex differences are not accounted for in the denominator, the crude birth rate does not represent a true probability of childbearing applicable to any individual member of that population. Because populations vary in their age and sex distributions, comparisons of crude birth rates of different populations are limited. Likewise, changes over time in the annual crude birth rates of a population may be due to changes in the age or sex composition of the population rather than due to changes in the fertility of the population.

A measure that more appropriately relates births to an approximation of the population at risk is the general fertility rate (GFR). The denominator is composed of women aged 15–44. Obviously, only women are "at risk" of childbearing. Although women younger than 15 or older than 44 may give birth, it is within these age bounds that most childbearing occurs.

$$GFR = \frac{\text{Number of live births during interval}}{\text{Average population during interval}} \times 1,000$$

The total fertility rate (TFR) is the sum of annual age-specific birth rates for women aged 10–49. Because these statistics are usually kept for 5-year age groups, the rate for each age group is multiplied by five before summing the rates to obtain the TFR. Not only does the TFR have the advantage of a more inclusive "at risk" population (10–49 rather than 15–44), but, because it is made up of age-specific rates, it is not influenced by the age distribution of the women in the population.

Another widely used summary of age-specific rates is the gross reproduction rate (GRR). The GRR is the same as the total fertility rate except that only female births are counted. The GRR can be quickly computed from the TFR by multiplying the TFR by the percentage of births that are female.

The net reproductive rate (NRR) differs from the GRR in that only those female births who will survive until reproductive age at current mortality rates are included in the rate. The calculations of TFR, GRR, and NRR are illustrated in Table 6.1.

A GRR of 1,000 signifies that if all the women born at the beginning of a generation survive through their reproductive period and as a group continue to give birth at this rate, they will exactly reproduce themselves. However, mortality before reproductive age will prevent complete replacement. An NRR of 1,000 means that each generation of women will just replace itself. A net rate of less than 1,000 indicates a potentially declining population, whereas an NRR greater than 1,000 signifies potential population increase.

Mortality Measures

Mortality describes the frequency of deaths over a period of time. These measures are among the most widely used statistics in epidemiology, partly because they are among the most accurately counted events in all of our health statistics.

The crude death rate represents the risk of dying for a randomly selected individual from the entire population of a designated area.

TABLE 6.1 Total, Gross, and Net Reproduction Rates: United States, 1981

Age Group in Years	Age-Specific Fertility Rates Per 1,000 Women	(x) Proportion of Females at Birth[a]	(=) GRR	(x) Proportion Surviving Females (1_x)[b]	(=) NRR
10–14	1.1	.488	.54	.9757	0.52
15–19	52.7	.488	25.72	.9743	25.05
20–24	111.8	.488	54.56	.9715	53.01
25–29	112.0	.488	54.66	.9680	52.91
30–34	61.4	.488	29.96	.9639	28.88
35–39	20.0	.488	9.76	.9581	9.35
40–44	3.8	.488	1.85	.9492	1.76
45–49	0.2	.488	0.09	.9363	0.08
Σ	363.0	.488	177.14	—	171.56
Σx5[c]	TFR = 1815	—	GRR = 885.7	—	NRR = 857.8

[a]The proportion of females at birth varies only slightly between age groups; the proportion of the total is an adequate figure to use.

[b]This data from current life tables. Use 1_x column and compute proportion of females surviving.

[c]TFR, GRR, and NRR: Values summed and multiplied by five (5) because age groups are in 5-year intervals.

Source: Statistical Abstract of the United States, 1985.

Computed from total deaths due to all causes and total population, it measures the decrease in a population due to death.

$$\text{Crude death rate} = \frac{\text{Total number of deaths during interval}}{\text{Total population}} \times 1{,}000$$

18   Specific death rates for any defined group within the population measure the risk of dying for any member of that group. They are computed from the number of deaths occurring in the defined group and the total number of persons in that group using the formula:

$$\text{Specific death rate} = \frac{\begin{array}{c}\text{Number of deaths}\\ \text{in specific group}\end{array}}{\text{Population of group}} \times 1{,}000$$

The groups for which specific death rates may be calculated may be defined by any characteristic or combination of characteristics provided that the characteristics are found both in the census and on death certificates. For example, a specific death rate might be calculated for white, divorced women between the ages of 40 and 49 if that suits the epidemiologist's purpose.

19   Perhaps the most epidemiologically important of all mortality rates are those that are specific as to cause of death. These rates represent the risk of death from a specific condition and may be either crude or specific—that is, the denominator may be either the total population or some specific population subgroup.

$$\text{Cause-of-death rate} = \frac{\begin{array}{c}\text{Number of deaths}\\ \text{due to a stated cause}\end{array}}{\text{Population at risk}} \times 100{,}000$$

$$\begin{array}{c}\text{Cause-of-death rate}\\ \text{for a specific}\\ \text{subgroup}\end{array} = \frac{\begin{array}{c}\text{Number of deaths}\\ \text{among a specified group}\\ \text{due to a stated cause}\end{array}}{\text{Population of group}} \times 100{,}000$$

Infant and Maternal Mortality Measures _____

The infant mortality rate traditionally has been considered of great importance in public health. It has been widely applied as an index of the general health of a community or nation, either to compare one to another or to study changes over time. As an index it has been found to be highly sensitive to variations in sanitary conditions, food resources, and medical care.

Infant mortality may be subdivided into two separate measures. Deaths during the first 27 days of life are known as *neonatal mortality*. Those occurring to infants less than 1 year of age but no less than 4 weeks old are termed *postneonatal mortality*. The death rate during the first year of life is higher than at any other age until old age. In less developed nations, the postneonatal mortality rate is only slightly less than the neonatal mortality rate. As nations become more developed, postneonatal deaths decline more than do neonatal deaths, widening the gap between the two rates.

As a general rule, the lower the infant mortality of a society is, the lower the proportion of those deaths that occur postneonatally. The higher the infant mortality rate, the higher the proportion of postneonatal deaths. The lower the infant mortality rate, the higher the ratio of neonatal to postneonatal deaths. This relatively consistent relationship suggests that postneonatal mortality is more related to the sort of causal variables associated with economic development, such as improvements in sanitation, nutrition, and medical care. Neonatal mortality, on the other hand, appears to be less affected by such variables and may be more often due to genetic causes or complications of the birth process.

$$\text{Infant mortality rate} = \frac{\text{Number of deaths under 1 year of age during year}}{\text{Number of live births during year}} \times 1{,}000$$

$$\text{Neonatal mortality rate} = \frac{\text{Number of deaths under 28 days of age during year}}{\text{Number of live births during year}} \times 1{,}000$$

$$\text{Postneonatal mortality rate} = \frac{\text{Number of deaths occurring from 28 days, up to but not over 1 year of age during year}}{\text{Number of live births during year}} \times 1{,}000$$

33   The infant mortality rate should be the sum of the neonatal and postneonatal mortality rates. However, in calculating the postneonatal mortality rate according to the formula given above, some degree of error is introduced, which decreases the precision of any such summing process. The degree of error is usually negligible and for most practical purposes can be discounted. Nevertheless, it is true that those infants who died during the neonatal period (the first 4 weeks after birth) were not, of course, "at risk" of dying again during the postneonatal period. Therefore, a more precise calculation of the postneonatal death rate would require that the number of neonatal deaths be subtracted from the denominator of the rate. This seldom-used but more precise formula is:

$$\text{Postneonatal death rate} = \frac{\begin{array}{c}\text{Number of deaths of infants}\\\text{more than 28 days old}\\\text{but less than 1 year old}\end{array}}{\begin{array}{c}\text{Number of live births that year}\\\text{minus number of neonatal deaths}\end{array}} \times 1{,}000$$

    There is another source of error in all of the infant mortality rates. In fact, they are not truly rates at all; they are only ratios. One of the essential elements of a rate is that all of the persons represented in the numerator must also be represented in the denominator. All of the infant mortality measures violate this principle. The problem is simply
34 that an infant may be born during one calendar year and die during the next while still less than 1 year old. For instance, if an infant born on December 31, 1987 dies on January 1, 1988, it is included in the numerator but not the denominator for the 1988 infant and neonatal mortality rates. Likewise, that infant is included in the denominator for the 1987 postneonatal death rate, although it was not actually at risk for postneonatal death in 1987.

35   A fetal death (or stillbirth) is one in which an infant is delivered dead. If the infant shows any sign of life after the delivery—such as pulsation of the umbilical cord or movement of the voluntary muscles—then it is considered a live birth followed by a neonatal death.

    The fetal mortality rate is intended as a measure of the risk of fetal death among all pregnancies carried beyond a specified period of gestation (usually 20 weeks). An alternate statistic, the fetal death ratio, relates fetal deaths to live births. Due to incomplete reporting and variations in reporting requirements, neither of these statistics is generally a good measure of the true risk of fetal death. Any conclusions based on these statistics should be approached with the greatest of caution.

$$\text{Fetal mortality rate} = \frac{\begin{array}{c}\text{Number of fetal deaths}\\\text{of specified period of gestation}\end{array}}{\begin{array}{c}\text{Number of live births}\\\text{plus number of fetal deaths}\\\text{of specified period of gestation}\end{array}} \times 1{,}000$$

$$\text{Fetal death ratio} = \frac{\begin{array}{c}\text{Number of fetal deaths}\\\text{of specified period of gestation}\end{array}}{\text{Number of live births}} \times 1{,}000$$

Perinatal mortality is a concept that combines fetal deaths with loss of life in early infancy. A majority of neonatal deaths arise from conditions established before delivery or from complications of the birth process itself. Similar causes are likely to be responsible for the loss of viable fetuses. Thus, combining the two into a single rate seems logical. It also eliminates discrepancies that may arise from the recording of live births as fetal deaths or vice versa.

A single definition of perinatal mortality has not yet been agreed on. There are two commonly used formulae, usually referred to by the designations *PMR* I and *PMR* II. There are arguments for the choice of each formula. The critical consideration is that the method used must always be specified. Any comparisons should only be made where the figures are all calculated by the same formula.

$$PMR\ \text{I} = \frac{\begin{array}{c}\text{Infant deaths under 7 days of age}\\\text{plus fetal deaths of 28-weeks gestation}\end{array}}{\begin{array}{c}\text{Number of live births}\\\text{plus fetal deaths of 28-weeks gestation}\end{array}} \times 1{,}000$$

$$PMR\ \text{II} = \frac{\begin{array}{c}\text{Infant deaths under 28 days of age}\\\text{plus fetal deaths of 20-weeks gestation}\end{array}}{\begin{array}{c}\text{Number of live births}\\\text{plus fetal deaths of 20-weeks gestation}\end{array}} \times 1{,}000$$

The maternal mortality rate reflects not only the quality of obstetrical care but also the general level of environmental and social health in the community. This statistic relates the number of childbirth-associated (puerperal) deaths to the number of live births during the same interval (usually 1 year). Technically this is a ratio, not a rate, because the numerator (mothers) is not included in the denominator (infants).

Live births are used in calculating this statistic because that is the way the data are recorded—a birth certificate for each infant rather than for each mother or each pregnancy. Live births, of course, do not represent all pregnancies at risk for maternal death. To arrive at such a denominator we would have to include fetal deaths as well. Given the unreliability of fetal death registrations, it has become customary not to bother.

$$\text{Maternal mortality rate} = \frac{\text{Number of deaths due to puerperal causes}}{\text{Number of live births}} \times 1{,}000$$

Adjusted Rates

If we were to conduct a study of mortality rates in relation to hair color, we might find that people with gray or white hair showed significantly higher mortality rates than persons with any other color hair. It would be unwise, however, to conclude that gray or white hair is causally related to high mortality. The problem, obviously, is that gray or white hair is often associated with old age and that the elderly have a higher annual death rate than the young.

This problem is known as *confounding.* The above example is a confounder because it is causally associated with both age and mortality. This makes it difficult to assess any possible effect of hair color on mortality. One way to do so would be to only compare persons of the same age—is hair color associated with mortality rates among 20-year-olds, for instance. The other way is to statistically adjust the data so as to eliminate the influence of age differences between the different hair color groups.

We experience exactly this same problem in many epidemiologic comparisons between groups or communities. It would not be surprising to learn that the crude death rate in St. Petersburg, Florida, with its large number of retirees, is greater than that in Gainesville, Florida, with its large number of University of Florida students. An older population is likely to have a higher death rate and (as will be discussed in Chapter 8) different morbidity rates than a younger population. In fact, age is almost always a confounding factor whenever two communities are compared. For this reason, such comparisons should always be made using age-adjusted rates.

Age-adjusted (standardized) rates are rates that have been statisti- 42
cally transformed into the rates that would exist in the communities
under comparison if both communities had the same age distribution. Adjusted rates may be calculated for natality and morbidity, 43
as well as for mortality. Rates may be adjusted, or standardized, not
only for age but also for other person factors, such as race and sex. The 44
most frequently used adjusted rates, however, are age-adjusted mortality rates. We will use such rates to illustrate the adjustment process. 45

For our example, we will take two hypothetical counties—Snow
County and Frost County. In 1960, the crude death rate in Snow County
was 15.3 per 1,000 population. The crude death rate in Frost County in
1960 was 6.7 per 1,000. The age distributions of the two populations
are found in Table 6.2. An examination of the table shows the age
distributions of the two counties to be quite different. The population of

TABLE 6.2   Age Distribution of the Population of Two Hypothetical Counties

Age Group in Years	Snow County		Frost County	
	Population	Distribution (Percent)	Population	Distribution (Percent)
<1	5,674	1.52%	4,597	2.90%
1–4	22,167	5.92	17,128	10.80
5–9	26,713	7.13	17,877	11.27
10–14	25,219	6.73	14,575	9.19
15–19	18,710	4.99	12,481	7.87
20–24	13,855	3.70	14,906	9.40
25–29	15,401	4.11	12,966	8.17
30–34	18,476	4.93	12,393	7.81
35–39	20,966	5.60	11,113	7.00
40–44	20,667	5.52	9,663	6.09
45–49	20,582	5.49	8,111	5.11
50–54	21,088	5.63	6,474	4.08
55–59	23,238	6.20	5,118	3.23
60–64	28,747	7.67	3,735	2.35
65–69	36,610	9.77	3,152	1.99
70–74	29,173	7.79	2,048	1.29
75–79	16,415	4.38	1,341	0.85
80–84	7,243	1.93	588	0.37
85+	3,721	0.99	357	0.23
Totals	374,665	100.00%	158,623	100.00%

Source: Ferrara, C. P. (1980). *Vital and health statistics.* Atlanta, GA: Centers for
Disease Control.

Snow County had a median age of 44 years, with 24.9 percent of the population over age 65. Frost County's population had a median age of 24 and only 4.7 percent of them were over age 65. Obviously, these age differences are likely to be responsible for much of the difference in the two counties' death rates.

Two traditional methods exist for the adjustment of rates. These are the *direct method* and the *indirect method*. More recently, a number of procedures have been developed using multiple linear regression, multiple logistic functions, or discriminant function analysis to adjust rates. These procedures are beyond the scope of this text. The interested reader is referred to Kahn (1983) for a detailed discussion of these methods.

Direct Adjustment

In the direct method of age-adjusting rates, the age-specific rates from the study populations are applied to a standard population to obtain the number of "expected deaths" for each age group. The expected deaths are those that would be expected to occur if the age distribution of the study population were the same as that of the standard population. Any population distribution can be used as a standard population. Among the most commonly chosen standard populations are the population of the United States, the population of the state in which both communities are located, or a hypothetical pooled population created by adding the two community populations together. For the purpose of this example, we will use the 1980 Census population of the U.S. as our standard population.

A necessary step for direct adjustment is the calculation of age-specific death rates for the two counties under study. The results of these calculations, using the general formula for specific death rates, are shown in Table 6.3.

Table 6.4 shows the calculations for direct adjustment of the rates. For each age group (first column), the standard population (second column) is multiplied by the age-specific death rate for each county (third and fourth columns). The result is entered into the fifth or sixth column, respectively. For example, the calculation for the expected number of infant deaths in Snow County is:

$$\text{Expected deaths} = \frac{22.8}{1,000} \times 3,612,000 = 82,353$$

TABLE 6.3 Population, Resident Deaths, and Death Rates by Age in Two Hypothetical Counties

Age Group in Years	Snow County			Frost County		
	Population in 1960	Deaths in 1960	Rate (per 1,000 Pop.)	Population in 1960	Deaths in 1960	Rate (per 1,000 Pop.)
<1	5,674	160	28.2	4,597	105	22.8
1–4	22,167	30	1.4	17,128	23	
5–14	51,932	30	0.6	32,452	21	0.6
15–24	32,565	26	0.8	27,387	39	1.4
25–34	33,877	47	1.4	25,359	48	
35–44	41,633	124	3.0	20,776	83	4.0
45–54	41,670	320	7.7	14,585	137	9.4
55–64	51,985	829	15.9	8,853	182	
65–74	65,783	1,901	28.9	5,200	204	39.2
75+	27,379	2,259	82.5	2,286	223	97.6
Totals	374,665	5,726	15.3	158,623	1,065	6.7

Source: Ferrara, C. P. (1980). *Vital and health statistics.* Atlanta, GA: Centers for Disease Control.

TABLE 6.4 Direct Method of Adjustment Mortality in Two Hypothetical Counties Using the 1980 U.S. Enumerated Population as Standard

Age Group in Years	Enumerated Standard Population (U.S. 1980) (in thousands)	(x) Age-Specific Death Rates (per 1,000 Population)		(=) Expected Deaths in 1960 U.S. Population Using County Age-Specific Rates	
		Snow County	Frost County	Snow County	Frost County
<1	3,612	28.2	22.8	101,858	82,354
1–4	12,736	1.4	1.3	17,830	16,557
5–14	34,942	0.6	0.6	20,965	20,965
15–24	42,487	0.8	1.4	33,990	59,482
25–34	37,082	1.4	1.9	51,915	70,456
35–44	25,634	3.0	4.0	76,902	102,536
45–54	22,800	7.7	9.4	175,560	214,320
55–64	21,703	15.9	20.6	345,078	447,082
65–74	15,581	28.9	39.3	450,291	612,333
75+	9,969	82.5	97.6	822,443	972,974
Totals	226,546	15.3	6.7	2,096,831	2,599,059
Adjusted rates	—	—	—	9.3	11.5

Adapted from: Ferrara, C. P. (1980). Vital and health statistics. Atlanta, GA: Centers for Disease Control.

Once all of the number of expected deaths has been calculated for each age group in each county, the column of figures can be summed to arrive at the total number of expected deaths for each county. An adjusted death rate can then be calculated by dividing the number of expected deaths by the population of the county and multiplying the quotient by 1,000. Although time consuming, this is a mathematically simple procedure. The use of computers, of course, eliminates the time-consuming aspect.

Indirect Adjustment

For direct adjustment it is necessary to know both the number of persons and the number of deaths in each age group for both counties. In some cases, however, the mortality by age group may not be available and therefore the direct method cannot be used. In other instances, some of the age group populations may be so small that a difference of only a few deaths would cause large fluctuations in age-specific rates, thus rendering direct adjustment misleading. These problems are avoided by use of the indirect method.

In the indirect method the age-specific death rates from a standard population are applied to the age distribution in the study populations—exactly the opposite of the direct method. In our example, we use the 1981 age-specific death rates for the U.S. population. The method is presented in Table 6.5.

Expected deaths are calculated as in the direct method. An index death rate is then calculated by summing the number of expected deaths for each county and dividing by the county's population, then multiplying by 1,000. Then for each county, calculate an adjusting factor by dividing the crude death rate for the standard population by that county's index death rate. Finally, multiply the crude death rate for each county by the adjusting factor for that county in order to arrive at an adjusted death rate. Although this process may seem complex on first examination, it is actually quite simple to perform. The only problem, again, is that it is a lengthy process, but this is solved by the use of a computer.

Whichever method of adjustment is used, the results are essentially the same. Once the influence of differing age distributions is eliminated, the adjusted death rate in Frost County turns out to be higher than in Snow County. Hopefully, this serves to illustrate the value as well as the methods of age adjustment. Further examples of rate adjustment can be found in Ferrara (1980)—illustrations of adjustment of natality and mortality rates, and adjustment for race, sex, and age.

TABLE 6.5 Indirect Method of Adjustment Mortality in Two Hypothetical Counties Using 1980 U.S. Age-Specific Death Rates as Standard

Age Group in Years	Death Rates (per 1,000 Pop.) (U.S. 1981)	Population		Expected Deaths in County Using U.S. Specific Rates	
		Snow County	Frost County	Snow County	Frost County
<1	11.4	5,674	4,597	65	52
1–4	0.6	22,167	17,128	13	10
5–14	0.2	51,932	32,452	10	6
15–24	0.6	32,565	27,387	20	16
25–34	0.8	33,877	25,359	27	20
35–44	1.6	41,633	20,776	67	33
45–54	4.1	41,670	14,585	171	60
55–64	9.3	51,985	8,853	483	82
65–74	21.4	65,783	5,200	1,408	111
75+	54.4	27,379	2,286	1,489	124
Totals	9.5	374,665	158,623	3,753	514
Index death rates	Expected deaths ÷ population × 1,000			10.02	3.24
Adjusting factors	Standard death rate ÷ index death rate			0.948	2.93
Crude rate				15.3	6.7
Adjusted rate	Adjusting factor × crude rate			14.5	19.6

Adapted from: Ferrara, C. P. (1980). *Vital and health statistics.* Atlanta, GA: Centers for Disease Control.

Recommended Reading _____

Ferrara, C. P. (1980). *Vital and health statistics: Techniques of community health analysis.* Atlanta, GA: Centers for Disease Control.

Kahn, H. A. (1983). *An introduction to epidemiologic methods.* New York: Oxford University Press. (Chapters 5 and 6.)

Metter, G. E. (1986). Cancer trends: Measures and limitations and their relevance to cancer in women. *Health Values, 10*(1), 41–44.

Zemach, R. (1984). What the vital statistics system can and cannot do. *American Journal of Public Health, 74,* 756–758.

CHAPTER 7

Measures of Disease and Disability

Although mortality figures are useful in the study of disease, they would give us a very distorted view of the frequency of many diseases if they were the only measures available. Fortunately, we have a number of useful statistics with which to measure disease and disability. These are referred to as *morbidity measures*. The most important of these are measures of the *prevalence* and *incidence* of disease.

Prevalence Measures

Prevalence—the proportion of the population suffering a disease—has already been introduced in the Prolog. This useful statistic may be categorized temporally into point prevalence, period prevalence, and lifetime prevalence.

Point prevalence is the proportion of persons suffering from a particular disease in a population at a given time. The most common use of point prevalence is as an estimate of the need for services in a community. It is also useful for identifying groups at high risk for having a disorder, and as an outcome measure for the evaluation of the effectiveness of prevention programs in reducing the burden of disease on the community.

Period prevalence is the proportion of the population suffering from a particular disease during a specified period of time. The numerator is arrived at by adding the number of prevalent cases at the beginning of the defined period to the incident cases (first or recurrent) that developed during the period. The denominator is the average population size during the period.

The average population as the denominator seems a simple thing to say but it is seldom possible to obtain. To calculate the average daily population for a period, it is necessary to have a record of the population on each day of that period. The daily population figures are then summed and divided by the total number of days in the period. There are very few populations for which daily population figures are available—populations such as schools, hospitals, or prisons. For other populations it is simply not possible to calculate an average population size to use as a denominator.

The standard textbook solution to this problem is to use the midinterval (usually midyear) population figure. Thus, the denominator for an annual prevalence rate would be the population on July 1. Unfortunately, populations are not much more likely to undergo a census on July 1 of each year than they are to undergo a daily census. In reality—no matter what most textbooks may say—the denominator for most period rates is simply the most recent decennial census figure.

Lifetime prevalence is the proportion of individuals in a population on a given day who have ever suffered from the disease of interest. Because those who die are not included in either the numerator or the denominator of the lifetime prevalence rate, it is sometimes called the proportion of survivors affected (PSA).

Lifetime prevalence differs from lifetime risk, which measures the probability of the disease occurring during the entire lifetime of a birth cohort and includes those deceased at the time of the study. Proportion of cohort affected (PCA) is a similar measure that takes as its numerator all members of a given cohort, living or dead, who have ever suffered the disease under study by the study date. The morbidity risk ratio (MRR) is an adjusted form of the PCA that has been corrected to adjust for mortality due to other causes in the cohort. Although these measures have some advantages over lifetime prevalence, they are more troublesome to calculate, requiring that the numbers of deceased be determined, that their medical history be ascertained in relation to the disease under study, and that their age at death be determined. Furthermore, these alternatives to lifetime prevalence often rely on doubtful sources of information—most often relying on the memories of relatives or friends.

Incidence Measures

11 Incidence is a dynamic or time-dependent quantity. Incidence can be expressed as an instantaneous rate—the rate of new cases on a given day—but is more often expressed with a unit of time attached—as in an annual incidence rate.

12 Incidence may also be differentiated into first incidence and total incidence. First incidence refers only to cases that are new cases, in the sense of being the first occurrence of the disorder in the lifetime of the subject. Total incidence includes those new cases plus new recurrences *13* in individuals who have recovered from previous attacks.

The accuracy of incidence rates is obviously highly reliant on the prompt identification of new cases. If new cases occurring during the interval under study are not diagnosed during that interval, they cannot be included in the numerator. On the other hand, if diagnosis is delayed, cases that actually had their onset before the interval under study may be inappropriately included in the numerator.

It might be hoped that these two sources of error would roughly cancel each other out, but, when the rates are based on self-reports or reports by family members, the problem of telescoping arises. Telescop-*14* ing is the tendency to add events into the inquired-about time period that actually occurred earlier. This common error of human memory often results in incidence being overestimated where self-report data is used. On the other hand, self-report data may result in the inclusion of cases that were self-medicated and would not otherwise have been recognized and included in the incidence rates.

15 Incidence represents a measure of the spread to new persons of the disease or condition under study. As such it is particularly relevant to the planning of primary and secondary prevention programs. In the search for causes, it is the correlation between incidence rates and suspected causal factors that is usually most indicative of causation.

Measures of Disability

16 A taxonomy of the consequences of disease or injury, known as the International Classification of Impairments, Disabilities, and Handicaps (ICIDH), has been developed by the World Health Organization. An impairment is defined in ICIDH as any loss or abnormality of psychological, physiological, or anatomical structure or function. Impairments thus represent disturbances at the organ level.

Disability, according to the ICIDH, is any restriction or lack of ability to perform an activity in the manner or within the range considered normal for a human being. Such a restriction or lack of ability may be either an acute or a chronic condition. A disability is the consequence of an impairment. The term *disability* represents disturbances at the person level.

It is often useful to measure the extent to which illness is restricting the daily lives of the population. Commonly used as measures of the levels of acute disability are rates of restricted-activity days and bed-disability days experienced during some time period (usually 1 year).

Restricted-activity days are those days on which an individual does not carry on all of his or her normal activities because of an illness. These are days when an individual may go to work but may avoid the more strenuous demands of the job and return home early. These are days when an individual attends classes but does not devote extra time to studying at the library, and so on. Bed-disability days are those days when an individual stays home sick in bed.

The ICIDH defines a handicap as a disadvantage for a given individual, resulting from a disability, that limits or prevents the fulfillment of a role that would be considered normal for that individual (given the individual's age, sex, social status, and so forth) in that individual's culture. The term *handicap* thus reflects interaction with and adaptation to the person's surroundings. It might be said to represent disturbance at the social level.

Recommended Reading

Ferrara, C. P. (1980). *Vital and health statistics: Techniques of community health analysis.* Atlanta, GA: Centers for Disease Control.

Kramer, M., von Korff, M., & Kessler, L. (1980). The lifetime prevalence of mental disorders: Estimation, uses and limitations. *Psychological Medicine, 10,* 429–439.

PART III

The Epidemiologic Distributions

I keep six honest serving-men
(They taught me all I know);
Their names are What and Why and When
And How and Where and Who.

> — *Rudyard Kipling,*
> *"The Elephant's Child," (1902)*

The lines of verse above are often quoted to would-be journalists and authors as advice on the essential elements of any story—who did what, and where, when, how and why was it done. In similar terms Peterson and Thomas (1978) define epidemiology as "The professional discipline concerned with describing health related phenomena in human populations, specifically HOW MUCH with respect to WHEN, WHERE, and WHO for the purpose of explaining WHY such phenomena occur and WHAT can be done about them" (p. xv).

Epidemiologists have traditionally described the distribution of diseases (or other health-relevant phenomena) in terms of person (who), place (where), and time (when). Knowledge of each of these distributions is not only of value in planning interventions for the prevention and control of disease but also can provide valuable clues to the causes of disease.

CHAPTER 8

Person Factors

Person factors are concerned with the question of who is affected by the disease or health condition under study. Diseases do not affect all groups of people to the same extent. Knowledge of these differences in disease rates between different groups of people is of obvious value in planning health services for a community.

Such knowledge may also lead to the formulation of causal hypotheses. For instance, observation of person factors gave rise to the hypothesis that cervical cancer may be caused, in part, by a viral agent that is spread venereally with men as nondiseased carriers. Cervical cancer is rare among nuns but occurs at a high rate among prostitutes, and is more common among poor women than among middle-class or wealthy women. It is more common among women who married early. Lower-class women and women who marry early have shown a tendency to have more numerous sex partners. Thus, high rates of cervical cancer seem to be associated with groups of women likely to have more numerous sex partners, suggesting that the disease might be spread venereally.

The principle person factors of interest to epidemiologists are age, gender, race, and socioeconomic status. In recent years there has been increasing interest in the factors of stress, lifestyle, and health behaviors.

Age

Age is the most powerful of the person factors. This is said to be so for two reasons: first, age affects the distribution of almost every disease or health condition; and second, age has a greater effect on most distributions than does any other person factor. This is true to such an extent that it is often impossible to detect the influence of any other factors until the influence of age has been eliminated through rate adjustment (see Chapter 6).

The influence of age can be plainly seen on crude death rates. Death rates are highest in the neonatal period (the first 28 days of life) and decline through the remainder of infancy. From the age of 1 on the age-specific death rates increase year by year, finally exceeding the infant death rate after late middle age.

Figure 8.1 shows the five leading causes of death for five different age groups. This illustrates to some extent the impact of age on the distributions of disease. The figure illustrates the fact that the greatest threats to the lives of infants are those associated with the birth process or birth defects, while these play a declining role in the mortality of children after their first birthday. Also reflected in Figure 8.1 is the fact that the principal threats to the lives of the young are various forms of violence—accidents, homicide, and suicide. We can also see the increasing importance of chronic disease as age increases.

The common childhood diseases (chickenpox, measles, mumps, and so on) are so-called because they occur primarily in childhood, with peak rates between the ages of 5 and 9 and only rarely occurring in persons over 20. Rubella (German measles) has its peak incidence between the ages of 15 and 20, rarely occurring before 10 or after 30. Sudden infant death syndrome, as the name implies, seems to occur only during the first few years of life.

Applying epidemiologic methods to the problem of crime, we find that persons aged 12–15 are at highest risk of becoming victims of theft. Persons aged 16–19 are at highest risk of becoming victims of violent crimes such as rape, robbery, and assault. The risk of being a victim of either theft or violence declines steadily with age after 24. Although the elderly worry a great deal about theft and violent crime, they are least likely to actually become victims. The elderly (aged 65 and over) are most likely to be victims of fraud or other "white-collar" crimes.

Gender

The disease risks of males and females are seldom the same. In some cases the differences in rates appear to be clearly rooted in anatomical and physiological differences between men and women. Men do not

Rank	Infants	1–14	15–24	25–64	65 and older
1	Prematurity	Accidents other than vehicular	Motor vehicle accidents	Heart disease	Heart disease
2	Birth associated	Motor vehicle accidents	Accidents other than vehicular	Cancer	Cancer
3	Congenital birth defects	Cancer	Suicide	Stroke	Stroke
4	Sudden infant death	Congenital birth defects	Homicide	Cirrhosis of liver	Influenza and pneumonia
5	Influenza and pneumonia	Influenza and pneumonia	Cancer	Accidents other than vehicular	Arteriosclerosis

Figure 8.1 Five Leading Causes of Death by Age Groups. (*Source:* National Center for Health Statistics.)

develop uterine cancer and women do not develop cancer of the scrotum. Breast cancer is far more common among women than among men but is more likely to be fatal in a man than in a woman.

In many cases the differences seem more likely to be due to differences between the lifestyles of men and women. For instance, lung cancer remained rare among women after it had become common in men; now with women smoking more, lung cancer has become the most common fatal cancer in women as it has been for years among men. Men suffer a higher rate of chronic handicap than do women, probably due at least in part to more male participation in dangerous sports such as football, males being more likely to hold hazardous jobs, and the higher auto accident rates for male drivers.

Age-specific death rates for males are higher than those for females. Even fetal death rates are higher for males than for females. Paradoxically, women report more frequent illnesses and higher rates of restricted-activity days and bed-disability days than do men. This remains true even when disability related to pregnancy or menstruation is eliminated.

Depression appears to be twice as common among women as among men. Women are more likely to attempt suicide than are men. On the other hand, men are more likely to actually succeed in killing themselves than are women.

Men are about twice as likely to be victims of violent crimes as are women. The one exception to this is rape, which occurs seven times as often to females as to males. Males are also at somewhat greater risk of being victims of theft than are women.

Race

Some racial differences in disease risk clearly are genetic in nature (e.g., the higher risk of sickle cell anemia in blacks). Likewise, the higher rates of Tay-Sachs Disease (a fatal metabolic disorder affecting the nervous system) are among Ashkenazic Jews.

Other racial differences, such as higher infant mortality and shorter life expectancy among nonwhites, may well be due to social, economic, or cultural factors rather than biological ones. No one knows whether genetic or social factors, or some mix of the two, explains the high incidence of hypertension among blacks or the higher rates of cancer and heart disease among whites. Despite civil rights advances in recent decades, nonwhites are still seriously disadvantaged in the U.S. economy and are far more likely to be poor than are whites. Thus, the influence of race is often confounded with that of socioeconomic status.

Socioeconomic Status

Socioeconomic status (commonly abbreviated SES) is an important factor in the distribution of most diseases. In general, the poor are more susceptible to disease than are the wealthy. The poor suffer higher rates of heart disease, cancer, diabetes mellitus, vision problems, venereal disease, and so on.

Faris and Dunham (1939) studied all psychiatric hospital admissions in the Chicago area for the period 1922–1934 and plotted prevalence rates based on the patients' place of residence at the time of admission. They found that the rates showed a regular increase from the more affluent suburbs to the inner-city slums. This pattern held for all diagnoses combined and, especially, for the diagnosis of schizophrenia. They concluded that poverty was a cause of schizophrenia and that the slums were the "breeding ground" of mental illness. This came to be known as the breeder hypothesis and was generally accepted for the next quarter-century.

The suggestion by Myerson (1940) that the mentally ill had merely "drifted" into the slums was widely ignored. Eventually, however, evidence accumulated that forced a reexamination of this alternate hypothesis. Warren Dunham (1965), one of the two originators of the breeder hypothesis, demonstrated in studies in Detroit that, although mental hospital admission rates showed this pattern when plotted based on residence at time of admission, the pattern disappeared when cases were plotted based on place of birth. In other words, it does appear that the mentally ill tend to drift into the slums rather than the slums giving rise to high rates of mental illness. Today the drift hypothesis is generally accepted.

The term *breeder hypothesis* is often used now for any hypothesis that poverty causes disease. Any such hypothesis should always be tested against its alternative drift hypothesis—that the disease made its victims poor. Of course, the reality may, in many cases, be that both are true—poverty raises one's risk of disease and disease plunges one deeper into poverty.

Maternal Age _____

Teenage mothers are customarily defined as being "high-risk pregnancies" by physicians and other health authorities. The evidence does
not seem to support our society's prejudice against teenage pregnancy.
Teenage mothers are not at higher risk of giving birth to a low-birth
weight infant than are older mothers of the same SES. Apgar scores,
which rate an infant's physical condition 1 minute after birth, are
inversely correlated with maternal age. That is, the younger the mother
(at least down to age 14), the healthier the baby is likely to be. In terms
of risk to the mother's life, mothers under the age of 15 have a risk of
puerperal death a little less than that of 35–40-year-old women. The
lowest maternal mortality rate is found in mothers aged 15–20 and
20–25 (almost identical rates), with increasing maternal mortality for
every 5-year age group thereafter.

Maternal age is closely related to the rates of a number of common
birth defects. The best known of these patterns is the association of
Down's Syndrome (Mongolism) with mothers over 30, as can be seen
from Figure 8.2. Older mothers are also more likely to have infants with
congenital malformations of the circulatory system, hydrocephalus,
cleft palate, or cleft lip. Infants born to mothers who are either under 20
or over 40 are at increased risk of club foot. Teenage mothers are also at
greater risk of having babies with extra fingers or toes (polydactyly).
Until recently it was argued that the father's age did not have any
similar influence. Recent studies suggest that paternal age may be as
important as maternal age as a predictor of birth defects. It appears
that fathers over age 30 are an even stronger risk factor for Down's
Syndrome than mothers over age 30.

Other person factors that may be of interest in the study of some
diseases include educational level, family size, parental deprivation (by
death or divorce), birth order, blood type, and structural body type.

Stress _____

Stress as a causal factor in disease has been the subject of increasing
speculation and research in recent years. Hull (1977), for instance,
found 329 research articles on the subject in 19 journals for the 10-year
period 1965–1974. Although the subject is clearly of great interest and

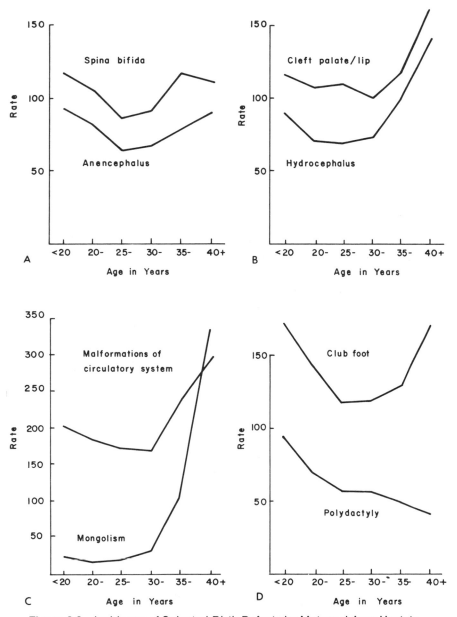

Figure 8.2 Incidence of Selected Birth Defects by Maternal Age: Upstate New York, 1950–1960 (cases per 100,000 live births). (*Source:* Gittelson, A. M., & Milham, S., Jr. (1965). Vital record incidence of congenital malformations in New York state. In J. V. Neel & M. W. Shaw (Eds.), *Genetics and the epidemiology of chronic diseases*. (USPHS Document No. 1163). Washington, DC: U.S. Government Printing Office, 134.)

apparently of great importance, research has been difficult due to the difficulties in defining and measuring an internal event or process such as stress.

One approach to the measurement of stress has been to ask subjects about their subjective experience of stress. Such questioning may take the direct form of asking subjects whether they are experiencing stress. Alternatively, it may take an indirect form in which an internal stress state is inferred from the subjects' reports of their mood and feeling, such as in the use of the HUMRRO Subjective Stress Scale, the State-Trait Anxiety Index, or the Mood Adjective Checklist. Such an approach assumes that individuals are aware of their own stress states and allows a substantial amount of potential bias to enter the measurement of stress. There is also the distinct possibility that the subjects' moods and feelings may have determinants other than stress that may prove inseparable using such an approach.

Another approach is the monitoring of presumed physiological correlates of stress. Measures of blood pressure, galvanic skin response, heart rate, respiratory rate, serum cholesterol, serum adrenaline, or skin temperature may be used as tracers indicating the experience and intensity of stress. Such methods place serious constraints on the study of stress. Population studies using such measures would be very difficult. Furthermore, we cannot assert that stress is the only cause of change in these tracer variables.

A highly popular approach has been to study external events, which are presumed to be stressors, and to assume that internal stress has resulted from these external events. Studies using this approach have examined such stressors as bereavement, divorce, surgery, loss of employment, beginning college, and combat military service. These studies, however, cannot address the subject of stress generally nor can they deal with the cumulative effects of a variety of smaller stressors.

Holmes and Rahe (1967) developed what has since become the most popular approach to the measurement of stress. Their Schedule of Recent Events (SRE) (mistakenly referred to in much of the literature as the Social Readjustment Rating Scale) is a list of 43 life events that require "social readjustment"—some change in one's way of life or attitudes. Each event on the SRE is assigned a value in terms of "life change units" (or LCUs) ranging from 11 for committing a minor violation of the law to 100 for the death of one's spouse. The LCU values of events occurring to an individual during the preceding year are summed to create a stress score. Scores less than 150 are considered normal; scores of 150–199 are labelled a mild life crisis; scores of

200–299, a moderate crisis; and scores of 300 or more, a major life crisis. The Schedule of Recent Events and the numerous scales based on it have become the most widely used method for the measurement of stress. There are, however, many unresolved issues in the use of this approach. For instance, should desirable life changes be counted along with aversive changes? How should weightings be assigned to the life events on the scale or should no weights be assigned? What sort of events should be included on the scale—only the major changes in life or the day-to-day hassles? For the present, these issues remain unresolved (Tausig, 1983; Kanner et al., 1981; Zimmerman, 1983).

Lifestyle and Behavior

A whole field of study of health behavior has grown since Parsons' (1951) description of sick-role behavior as a sociological phenomenon. Kasl and Cobb (1966a; 1966b) subsequently distinguished illness behavior and health behavior from sick-role behavior. Baric (1969) added the concept of at-risk behavior. The multitude of behavioral descriptors has grown since that time. In an attempt to summarize and lend order to the field, Kolbe (1983) has identified nine distinguishable, although not necessarily mutually exclusive, types of health-related behavior: wellness behavior, preventive health behavior, at-risk behavior, illness behavior, self-care behavior, sick-role behavior, family planning behavior, parenting health behavior, and health-related social action. Although behaviors in any of these categories may be of epidemiologic interest, the at-risk behaviors, such as smoking and excessive drinking, and the preventive health behaviors, such as exercise and dieting, have been most subject to epidemiologic investigation.

Probably the most influential work in this area has been that originating from the Human Population Laboratory's Alameda County Study, commonly referred to as the Breslow and Belloc Study after its two principal investigators (Berkman & Breslow, 1983). This study examined the mortality over a 9-year period and the self-reported health status of 6,928 persons aged 30–69 in relation to seven health practices and a measure of social support. Five of the health practices were found to be significant predictors of mortality. Persons who had reported only one or none of these five practices were 3.5 times more likely to have died during the 9-year follow-up period than were those who had reported three to five of the practices.

Stating them in a positive fashion, it was found that the risk of dying was significantly less in persons who:

1. were physically active
2. did not smoke
3. drank alcohol in moderation or not at all
4. were not obese
5. slept 7–8 hours per night.

Two other practices—eating breakfast every day and eating meals at regular times without snacking in between—were not found to be related to mortality. The same five practices were found to be significant predictors of self-reported health status. Despite the lack of evidence that the two eating related practices had any effect on health, all seven practices are widely believed to have been substantiated in this study and have been included in many prescriptions for a healthy lifestyle.

Subsequent analysis examined the social networks of the subjects in relation to mortality. Four types of social relationships were considered in this study: (1) marriage, (2) contacts with close friends and relatives, (3) church involvement, and (4) involvement in nonchurch groups. It was found that the most socially isolated men had an age-adjusted death rate 2.3 times higher than men with the strongest social networks. For women, the death rate among the socially isolated was 2.8 times that among those with the strongest social connections. Social networks and health practices appeared to be independently, and about equally, related to mortality.

Also worthy of special note is the concept of "Type A" behavior pattern (or coronary-prone behavior pattern) developed by Meyer Friedman (1984) and his colleagues. Type A behavior is characterized by a chronic sense of time urgency, high achievement motivation, competitiveness, devotion to job and career, aggressiveness, hostility, and impatience. Persons characterized by the absence of these traits are said to display Type B behavior pattern. A growing body of research confirms a strong association between Type A behavior and subsequent cardiovascular disease (Jenkins, 1976).

Epidemiologic studies have been conducted on a wide range of health behaviors, sometimes supporting causal hypotheses and other times disconfirming them. It seems likely that this area of study will increase in the future.

Recommended Reading ————————————————————

Kasl, S., & Cobb, S. (1966). Health behavior, illness behavior and sick-role behavior. *Archives of Environmental Health, 12,* 246–266.

Page, H. S., & Asire, A. J. (1985). *Cancer rates and risks* (3rd ed.). DHHS Publication (NIH) 85–691. Washington, DC: Government Printing Office.

Mechanic, D. (1979). The stability of health and illness behavior: Results from a six-year follow up. *American Journal of Public Health, 69,* 1142–1145.

CHAPTER 9

Place Factors

Place factors describe where diseases or health conditions occur. The differing rates for different places are important to know. Such knowledge is essential for the purposes of local and regional health planning and can be critical in monitoring the spread of any new disease threat.

Place factors may also provide clues to causation. It was the study of geographical distribution of mottled teeth (tooth enamel with brown patches) that led to the discovery that this condition was caused by drinking water with extraordinarily high levels of naturally occurring fluoride. Further study revealed that the prevalence of this condition, now known as fluorosis, was inversely related to the prevalence of tooth decay (dental caries). The subsequent discovery that fluoride could protect against tooth decay at concentrations too low to cause fluorosis has given rise to water fluoridation and hope for the eventual eradication of dental caries.

A caveat must be given, however, about drawing conclusions from place factor studies. Although they can be useful in suggesting causal hypotheses, as they did in the preceding example, the proof of a causal hypothesis requires the types of analytic studies discussed in Part IV of this text. Place factor studies are subject to what is known as the "ecological fallacy," in which correlations drawn from group data may produce results contrary to those that would be derived from correlations for individuals (Robinson, 1950; Scheuch, 1966). The same problem may hold true for person factor studies.

We might imagine a place where half the population is over 7 feet tall. The other half of the population is of normal height but suffers from vertigo (chronic dizziness). No one over 7 feet tall, in this peculiar place, ever suffers from vertigo. Nevertheless, if we looked at statistics for this total population in comparison with a more typical population in terms of average height and prevalence of vertigo, we would find a correlation between height and vertigo. The false conclusion that height causes vertigo (or vice versa) would, in this example, be a case of the ecological fallacy.

Another example is to compare the average height of a group of men to that of a group of women. If the men are a group of jockeys and the group of women is a basketball team, we might draw the wrong conclusion about which sex tends to be taller.

So long as we remember that descriptive epidemiology can only suggest hypotheses—not prove them—evidence such as place factors can be of great value to the epidemiologist. The place factors of greatest interest to epidemiology fall into four categories: international comparisons, intranational comparisons, urban–rural comparisons, and local comparisons.

International Comparisons

In international comparisons we contrast the rates of a health-relevant phenomenon in two or more nations. Such comparisons are a continuing concern of national health authorities responsible for quarantine and immunization requirements for international travelers. Cholera, for instance, is very rarely encountered in the Western hemisphere (especially in the United States or Canada) or Northern Europe, but is a serious problem in much of South Asia (especially India and Indonesia), Africa, and the Eastern Mediterranean region.

Very substantial differences in prevalence of diseases often exist between nations. Such differences may suggest useful causal hypotheses about the diseases in question. Japan, for example, has the highest mortality rate due to stomach cancer of any developed nation, while the United States has the lowest (about one-sixth that of Japan). On the other hand, Japan has the lowest mortality rate among developed nations for breast cancer, and the United States (with a rate more than four times as high) has about the median rate for developed nations. When Japanese move to the U.S., their risk for the two cancers becomes closer to the U.S. rates and second generation Japanese–Americans have about the same risk as all other Americans. Obviously,

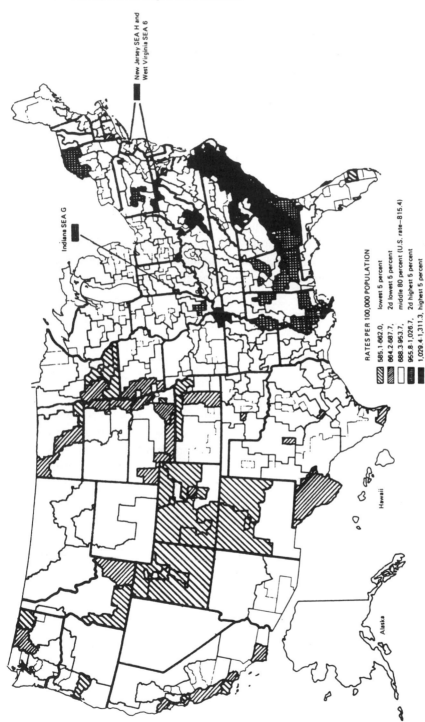

Figure 9.1 Mortality Due to Cardiovascular Diseases in White Males Aged 35–74, by State Economic Areas: United States, 1968–1972. (*Source:* Mason, T. J., Fraumeni, J. F., Jr., Hoover, R., & Blot, W. J. (1981). *An atlas of mortality from selected causes.* Washington, DC: U.S. Government Printing Office.)

RATES PER 100,000 POPULATION

585.1–662.0, lowest 5 percent
664.2–687.7, 2d lowest 5 percent
688.3–953.7, middle 80 percent (U.S. rate—815.4)
955.8–1,026.7, 2d highest 5 percent
1,029.4–1,311.3, highest 5 percent

New Jersey SEA H and West Virginia SEA 6

Indiana SEA G

Hawaii

Alaska

there are differences between the environments (physical, biological, or social) of Japan and the United States that are causally important to these two types of cancer. What those relevant differences are is a subject of considerable research at present.

Intranational Comparisons

In making intranational comparisons we contrast the rates in different parts of the same nation—different regions, states, etc. For instance, a number of north–south gradients have been identified, such as those in multiple sclerosis, violent crime, and alcoholism. For states in the United States, the mortality rates for multiple sclerosis tend to increase the farther north the state is. The same general pattern is found for MS mortality rates for major U.S. cities. Rates of violent crime (murder, rape, armed robbery, and aggravated assault) tend to increase as you look further south. Alcoholism was at one time reported to have a north–south gradient with highest rates in the north but more recent studies no longer show this pattern. Cardiovascular disease shows something of an east–west gradient with all but two of the areas with lowest mortality rates being west of the Mississippi River while only one of the areas with highest mortality is so located—that being the Bootheel region of Missouri just west of the Mississippi; see Figure 9.1.

Intranational patterns do not necessarily follow north–south or east–west gradients. Good examples are provided by two fungal infections of the human respiratory system—coccidioidomycosis and histoplasmosis. Coccidioidomycosis thrives in hot, arid conditions and occurs mainly in the southwest of the United States. Histoplasmosis, on the other hand, thrives in humid conditions and is found mainly along the inland river valleys of the Mississippi, Missouri, and Ohio rivers and their tributaries; see Figure 9.2.

Viral hepatitis has its highest incidence in the western and northeastern states. A high incidence of Rocky Mountain spotted fever is, not surprisingly, found in the Rocky Mountain region while another area of high incidence is in the southern Appalachian Mountains region. The prevalence of child abuse has been found to be highest in the midwest and lowest in the south. Areas with the highest mortality due to breast cancer are in the northeastern and east–north central states while the areas with lowest mortality are all in either the south or west of the Mississippi; see Figure 9.3.

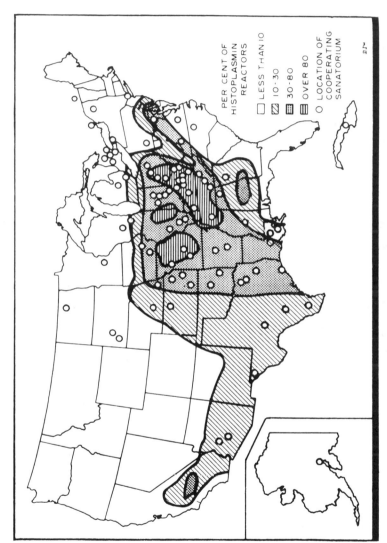

Figure 9.2 Prevalence of Histoplasmin Sensitivity: United States, 1962. (*Source:* Furcolow, M. L., et al. (1962). Serological evidence of histoplasmosis in sanatoriums in the U.S. *Journal of the American Medical Association, 180,* p. 110. Copyright 1962, American Medical Association.)

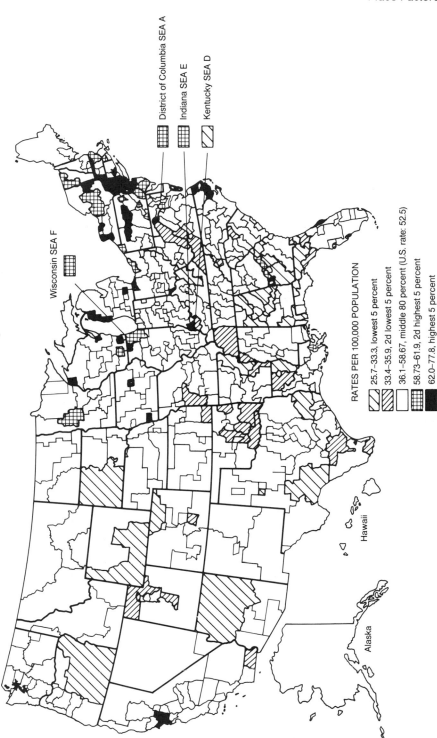

Figure 9.3 Mortality Due to Breast Cancer Among White Women Aged 35–74, by State Economic Areas: United States, 1968–1972. (*Source:* Mason, T. J., Fraumeni, J. F., Jr., Hoover, R., & Blot, W. J. (1981). *An atlas of mortality from selected causes.* Washington, DC: U.S. Government Printing Office.)

RATES PER 100,000 POPULATION

25.7–33.3, lowest 5 percent
33.4–35.9, 2d lowest 5 percent
36.1–58.67, middle 80 percent (U.S. rate: 52.5)
58.73–61.9, 2d highest 5 percent
62.0–77.8, highest 5 percent

District of Columbia SEA A
Indiana SEA E
Kentucky SEA D
Wisconsin SEA F

Hawaii

Alaska

Urban–Rural Comparisons

Comparing the rates of health-relevant phenomena found in urban areas to those in rural areas can be of great epidemiologic significance. It can also present serious methodological problems. To begin with, there is the problem that political boundaries do not match up with urban–rural differences—urbanicity does not end at the city limits. More difficult is the fact that there is no universally accepted definition of what is urban and what is rural. Within the context of southern Illinois, Carbondale (population 29,000) is considered urban, while compared to Chicago it is distinctly rural. Even greater confusion is added by suburbs, which are usually counted as urban but sometimes have been counted as rural, and which are, in fact, distinctly different from either one as health environments.

The generally accepted definition is that rural refers to open country and places or towns with less than 2,500 inhabitants unless they are part of the closely settled suburbs of metropolitan cities. Urban refers to: (1) cities with 50,000 or more inhabitants; (2) the closely settled areas around such cities (which are sometimes called "urbanized areas" rather than urban); and (3) towns with at least 2,500 inhabitants that are outside metropolitan areas.

It has long been noted that rates of admissions to mental hospitals were higher from predominantly rural counties than from predominantly urban counties. Such admissions rates may be a misleading indicator of the true incidence of mental disorder. To draw conclusions about the true levels of disease in a community based on the number of clinical cases is usually a mistake. The observed higher admissions rates from rural counties could reflect a lesser tolerance for abnormal behavior. The lower rates for urban areas might be due to the wider range of alternatives to hospitalization available in the urban setting.

Dohrenwend and Dohrenwend (1971) reviewed the epidemiologic evidence from nine studies of urban–rural differences in mental illness and found the evidence to be contradictory—one study showing the highest rates in rural areas, one showing no difference, and the remainder showing higher rates in urban areas. Their examination of the evidence suggests that the prevalence of psychoses is higher in rural areas while that of neuroses is higher in urban areas. Because the milder neuroses are more common than the more severe illness of the psychoses, total rates averaged out to a higher prevalence for urban areas.

Srole (1972; 1978) argues that many of the urban places in the studies reviewed by the Dohrenwends were not urban by contemporary American standards. Srole mustered evidence from several sources to support his view that mental illness in general is more prevalent in rural areas than urban. His data show a clear inverse relationship between population size and mean level of psychiatric symptomatology in communities. Edgerton et al. (1970) and Schwab et al. (1974) found a higher prevalence of mental illness in the rural populations of North Carolina and Florida, respectively, while Keller et al. (1979) found that in the northeastern states suicide rates were significantly higher for rural areas. During the 1960s Selective Service rejection rates for psychosis were 3.1 per 1,000 for urban draftees and 4.5 per 1,000 for rural draftees, while the rejection rates due to neurosis were 37 per 1,000 urban and 44 per 1,000 rural (Derr, 1973). The weight of the evidence, thus, seems to support Srole's view that mental illness in general is at higher incidence in rural areas.

Rural areas also show higher rates of accidents, heart disease, skin cancer, and chronic illnesses in general. Urban areas show higher rates of venereal disease, most of the common infectious diseases, and cancer of most sites. In the 1960s urban areas showed far higher rates of drug abuse and illicit drug use than did rural areas. Today there is almost no difference in these rates except for heroin addiction, which remains primarily a problem of a few big cities.

Local Comparisons

Local comparisons do not simply mean any comparative study done locally. Much more specifically, they refer to a study in which the locations of individual cases are plotted on a map along with the locations of various other factors thought to have possible causal significance.

This technique was first used by John Snow (1855) in his famous studies of the causation of cholera. During the 1854 cholera epidemic in London, Snow marked on a map (Figure 9.4) the location of the place of residence of every person who died of cholera. He also marked on the map suspected sources of the contagion. His map showed that a majority of the persons who died of cholera lived closer to the Broad Street pump than they did to any other water source, indoor plumbing not existing in the neighborhood. He was able to show that the Broad

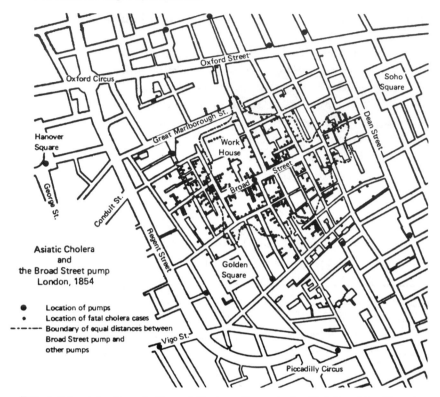

Figure 9.4 John Snow's Map of Cholera Cases in the Vicinity of the Broad Street Pump, London, 1854. (*Source:* Snow, J. (1936). *Snow on cholera.* New York: The Commonwealth Fund.)

Street pump was contaminated with human feces from a nearby privy. After he removed the handle from the pump, the epidemic ended. The term *local comparisons* refers to this technique of plotting cases on a map along with possible sources of the disease.

Another example of this technique involves an epidemic of infectious hepatitis among the children in a small Connecticut elementary school. Because cases did not occur among children in the same community who attended a Catholic school, the source of the epidemic was identified as being at the public school. Only children in the 3rd–6th grades had developed the disease, although children of all ages rode together on the school buses and ate the same food in the cafeteria. Once the cases were marked on a map (Figure 9.5) it became obvious that it was the location of their classroom on the west rather than on the east side of the building, and not their age, which explained why some children caught the disease and others did not. Children were apparently catching infectious hepatitis from the water at the school

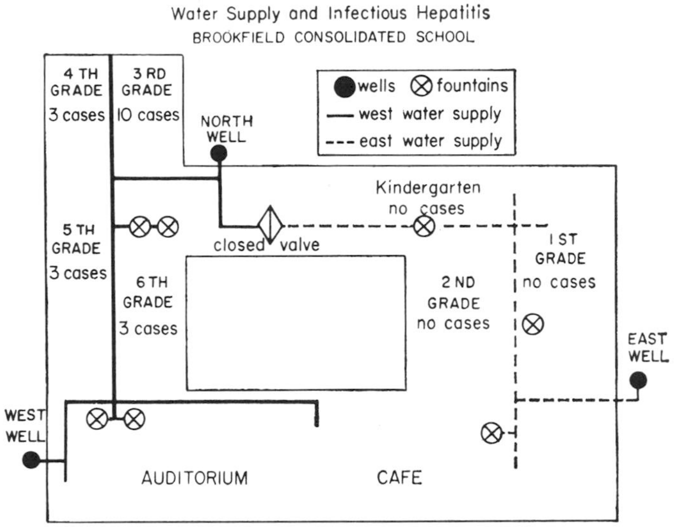

Water Supply and Infectious Hepatitis
BROOKFIELD CONSOLIDATED SCHOOL

Figure 9.5 Local Comparison of Water Supply and Cases of Infectious Hepatitis: Elementary School in Connecticut, 1960. (*Source:* Rindge, M. E., et al. (1962). Infectious hepatitis: Report of an outbreak in a small Connecticut school, due to water-borne transmission. *Journal of the American Medical Association, 180*, p. 36. Copyright 1962, American Medical Association.)

drinking fountains. Water from either the north or west well must have been contaminated. The end of the school year brought the epidemic to an end in this case before the epidemiologists could trace it to its source.

Recommended Readings

Howe, G. M. (1963). *National atlas of disease mortality in the United Kingdom (1954–1958)*. London: Nelson.

Hunter, J. M. (Ed.). (1974). *The geography of health and disease*. Chapel Hill: University of North Carolina.

Hutt, M. S. R., & Burkitt, D. P. (1986). *The Geography of Non-Infectious Disease*. New York: Oxford University Press.

Mason, T. J., McKay, F. W., Hoover, R., Blot, W. J., & Fraumeni, J. F. Jr. (1976). *Atlas of cancer mortality for U.S. counties, 1950–69* [DHEW Publication No. (NIH) 75–780]. Washington, DC: U.S. Government Printing Office.

McGlashan, N. D. (Ed.). (1977). *Medical geography: Techniques and field studies*. London: Methuen.

United Hospital Fund of New York, Division of Research, Analysis & Planning. (1985). *New York City community health atlas*. New York: United Hospital Fund of New York.

CHAPTER 10

Time Factors

Time factors deal with the when of disease occurrence. Knowledge of the changes over time in rates of disease can be of great value in predicting future disease experience, in assessing the impact of interventions, and in suggesting causal hypotheses.

The association between lung cancer and cigarette smoking was initially suggested by the similarity between the increasing popularity of cigarette smoking (a relatively uncommon practice a century ago in America) and the increasing mortality due to lung cancer (a rare form of cancer a century ago). False hypotheses, of course, may also be suggested by the same type of data. When it was observed that the numbers of diagnosed cases of hyperkinesis (now known as attention deficit disorder) showed a steady increase after World War II, which closely paralleled the increase in the number of new food additives approved in that period, this correlation suggested the hypothesis that hyperkinesis was caused by an allergy to some or all of those additives. Experimental tests of this hypothesis have since shown it to be false. Actually, the increase in number of diagnosed cases was probably largely due to increasing awareness of hyperkinesis, which was only newly recognized as a diagnostic label after World War II.

The time factors most often of interest in epidemiology are secular trends, seasonal variation, cyclic variation, and point epidemics.

Secular Trends

The word *secular* is most often used in the sense of "nonreligious," as in secular authorities or secular schools, but it also has a second

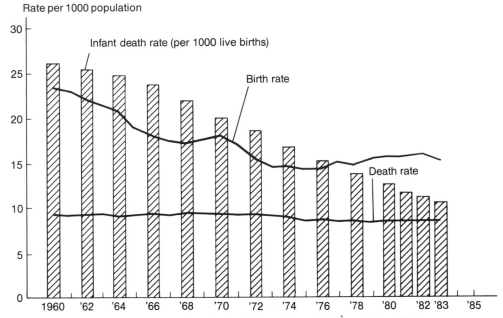

Figure 10.1 Secular Trends in Birth and Death Rates: United States, 1960–1983. (*Source: Statistical Abstract of the United States, 1985.*)

meaning, which is "coming or observed once in an age—once a century or once a decade—or extending over a long period of time." A secular trend, thus, is a pattern of continuous shift in rates in one direction over a long period of time—10 years or more. For instance, if we examine the age adjusted death rates in the United States from 1960 through 1983, as shown in Figure 10.1, we see a consistent downward trend over a quarter-century. In fact, this trend has been true for most of this century.

Trends in specific mortality rates for selected causes of death are shown in Figure 10.2. As can be seen from this figure, the secular trends for mortality due to stroke, influenza/pneumonia, and accidents (other than motor vehicle) have shown a steady decline throughout the century. Heart disease mortality increased until nearly midcentury and has been declining since then. Cancer has been increasing throughout this century. Motor vehicle accidents, on the other hand, show no consistent trend since they began being recorded in the 1920s, despite faster cars, new safety features, speed limit changes, or seat belts.

Rate per 100,000 population

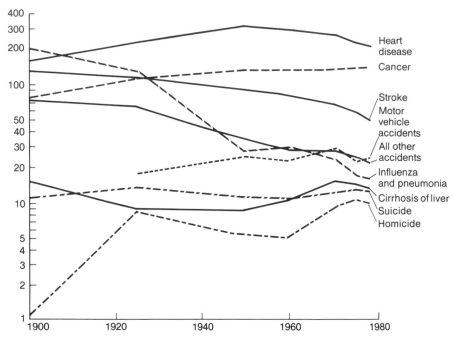

Note: The selected years are 1900, 1925, 1950, 1960, 1970, 1975, and 1978

Figure 10.2   Secular Trends in Age-Adjusted Death Rates from Selected Causes During Selected Years 1900–1978. (*Sources:* DHHS. (1979). *Healthy people: The Surgeon General's report on health promotion and disease prevention*; NCHS. (1956). *Special report on diabetes*, Vol. 43, No. 12; NCHS. (1956). *Vital statistics special report*, Vol. 43, No. 3.)

As can be seen from Figure 10.3, most of the common childhood infectious diseases show downward secular trends. Generally, downward trends since 1950 are shown for measles (rubeola), German measles (rubella), mumps, whooping cough (pertussis), diphtheria, and polio.

Seasonal Variation

Seasonal variation (or seasonal cyclicity) refers to changes in disease patterns that conform to a regular seasonal pattern. A peak of highest incidence occurs during one season and a trough of lowest incidence occurs in another season (usually about 6 months after the peak) year after year. We are all aware that the common cold and influenza are

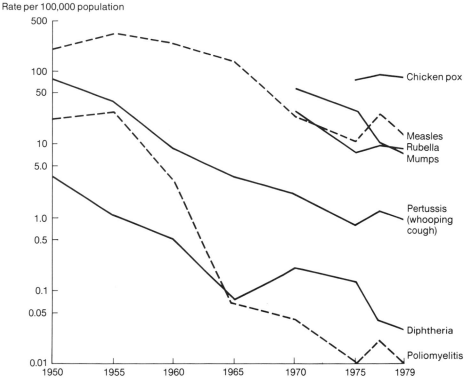

Figure 10.3 Secular Trends in Reported Incidence of Childhood Diseases During Selected Years 1950–1979. (*Sources:* CDC. *Morbidity and Mortality Weekly Report*, September 1979 and September 1980.)

most common in the winter and relatively rare in the summer, and that hay fever strikes from spring through early fall but not after the first heavy frost. Many of the seasonal patterns of disease are well recognized if not well understood.

Many of the common infectious diseases of childhood are seasonal with very low rates in the summer, rising in the fall to peaks in winter or spring. The primary reason for this pattern is the traditional American school year. Measles, mumps, chickenpox, and so on spread among children most readily when a lot of children are brought together in close proximity. Of course, this happens most notably in school and childhood infectious diseases are most often acquired at school. During the traditional summer vacation children rarely gather in such large and diverse groups and thus suffer low rates of infectious illness.

Aseptic meningitis is a nonbacterial (often an amoeba) infection of the meninges, the tough membranes that surround and protect the brain. This infection is most often acquired by swimming in non-chlorinated water. In most parts of the United States, swimming in ponds and streams is a summertime activity only. Thus, aseptic meningitis shows seasonal variation with the highest rates in late summer and lowest rates in midwinter.

Encephalitis, malaria, and yellow fever show a similar pattern of high incidence in summer and low incidence in winter. Here, however, the seasonal pattern is due to the fact that the infectious agents for these diseases are usually carried by mosquitoes. Because the vector is seasonal, the disease is seasonal.

Seasonal variation is not restricted to infectious diseases. Mental retardation, for instance, occurs more frequently among children born in the winter and least frequently among those born in the summer. Seasonal variation has also been reported for a number of common birth defects, such as cleft palate and spina bifida.

Tradition has ascribed a high incidence of suicide to the period around Christmas. When actual suicide rates are examined, however, it is found that December has the lowest suicide rate of any month. Suicides show a seasonal variation with higher rates in the spring and summer and lower rates in the fall and winter.

Cyclic Variation

Cyclic variation (sometimes called secular cyclicity) refers to repeated patterns of peaks and troughs in incidence rates, like those in seasonal variation, over a period of years rather than within a year. For example, in unimmunized populations measles tend to occur at high incidence every 3rd year. Likewise, hepatitis A has a peak incidence every 7 years.

The cycles in measles, hepatitis A, and a number of other infectious diseases are apparently due to the continuous exhaustion and replacement of susceptibles in a relatively stable population. During a peak year most of the susceptible persons in the community catch the disease. The following year most of the population has developed an immunity and only a few susceptibles remain. Even these susceptibles are protected to a degree by the fact that most of the people around them are immune.[1] With each passing year, the ratio of susceptibles to

---

[1] This partial protection afforded by a high percentage of immune persons in the community is known as herd immunity.

immunes rises until there are enough susceptibles in the community to support another major epidemic.

Point Epidemics

Point epidemics present a different type of time pattern. A point epidemic refers to a sudden rise in incidence that reaches a peak and then declines almost as rapidly. A point epidemic is so called, in part, because its origin can usually be traced to a particular point in time— when an infected person entered the community, when a contaminated meal was served, when the local water supply was contaminated, and so forth. The name also may derive, in part, from the characteristic shape of the epidemic curve that, as seen in Figures 10.4 and 10.5, is roughly shaped like a point.

Point epidemics are frequently encountered by epidemiologists. In fact, point epidemics are what we usually mean when we speak of an epidemic. Epidemics of food poisoning are a common concern of local public health authorities. Many infectious diseases show secular trend, cyclic variation, seasonal variation and point epidemics.

Although point epidemics are usually associated with infectious disease, there are cases where noninfectious illness occurs in point epidemics. For instance, the unplanned discharge of toxic chemicals

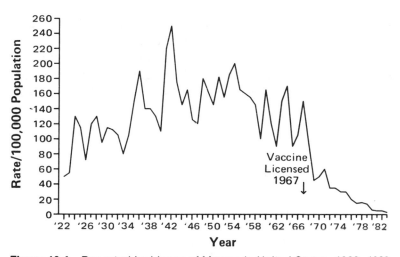

Figure 10.4 Reported Incidence of Mumps in United States, 1922–1983. (*Source:* National Center for Health Statistics, 1986.)

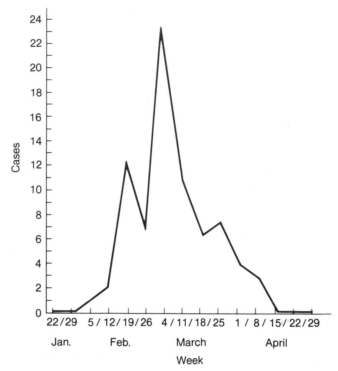

Figure 10.5 A Point Epidemic of Measles Cases by Week of Onset: Hobbs, New Mexico, 1984. (*Source: Mortality and Morbidity Weekly Reports*, Feb. 1, 1985.)

resulting in the contamination of air, water, or food may result in illness that will show the pattern of a point epidemic. Likewise, a point epidemic of leukemia has occurred in the populations of Hiroshima and Nagasaki following the atomic bomb blasts that ended World War II—a point epidemic in which the increase and subsequent decrease occurred over years instead of days.

Recommended Readings

Magnus, K. (Ed.). (1982). *Trends in cancer incidence*. New York: McGraw-Hill.
Office of Disease Prevention and Health Promotion, U.S. Department of Health and Human Services. (1981). Health status trends. In *Prevention '80* (Chapter 2). Washington, DC: U.S. Government Printing Office.

PART IV

Epidemiologic Research

Why are we taught that we can gain insight and the experience of beauty only through art, when this is but a limited and second-hand representation of the infinitely deeper experience to be gained by direct observation of the world around us? For such observation to become significant it must be made in the light of knowledge. The sense of wonder and excitement to be derived from watching the way an insect's wing functions, or an amoeba divides, or a foetus is formed comes in its greatest intensity only to those who have been given the opportunity to find out how these things happen.

— *James Burke (1978, p. 295)*

The next four chapters address the methods used in epidemiology to discover how and why things occur. This is often referred to as analytic epidemiology as distinguished from the preceding six chapters that were concerned with descriptive epidemiology.

The most powerful research strategy in epidemiology or any science is the experimental method as discussed in Chapter 11. An experiment provides firm evidence for or against any causal hypothesis so tested. Experimental methods, however, cannot always be applied to every study; therefore, quasiexperimental methods must often be substituted for the experimental method.

In epidemiology the two most commonly used quasiexperimental methods are the prospective cohort study and the case-control study. The prospective cohort study, as discussed in Chapter 12, can provide moderately firm evidence of causation. A case-control study, as discussed in Chapter 13, can only provide evidence which is strongly suggestive but not firm.

Chapter 14 discusses the application of analytic methods to the practical task of investigating an epidemic or outbreak. This is often referred to as field epidemiology.

121

CHAPTER 11

Experimental Studies

In the fifth century B.C., Judah was conquered by the Babylonians under King Nebuchadnezzar. The Jews had proven difficult to rule for previous conquerors, so Nebuchadnezzar took the precaution of taking hostages. Young men from the leading families of Judah were taken back to Babylon. As long as their families remained loyal to Nebuchadnezzar, they were to be well treated and would be taught the language and culture of the Babylonians.

Nebuchadnezzar ordered that the hostages were to be fed the same meat and served the same wine that was served to himself. Among the hostages was young Daniel, who was upset that he was to be fed nonkosher food and wine. He asked to be allowed to eat food prepared according to Jewish traditions but Melzar, the palace eunuch who had charge of the prisoners, was afraid to allow this. If the king were to find that one of his hostages was malnourished he would be angry and the eunuchs might pay with their heads. Daniel pleaded with Melzar to

'Prove thy servants, I beseech thee, ten days; and let them give us pulse to eat, and water to drink. Then let our countenances be looked upon before thee, and the countenance of the children that eat of the portion of the king's meat: and as thou seest, deal with thy servants.'

So he consented to them in this matter, and proved them ten days. And at the end of ten days their countenances appeared fairer and fatter in flesh than all the children which did eat the portion of the king's meat. Thus Melzar took away the portion of their meat, and the wine that they should drink; and gave them pulse. (Daniel, Ch. 1)

Thus we find the first account of the experimental method in the Old Testament.

New Names for the Experimental Method _____

Experiments provide the strongest possible evidence of causation. This is so much so that where sound experimental evidence exists, scientists will usually regard all other evidence as superfluous and meaningless. It has been said, with little exaggeration, that an experiment is for the scientist what a voice from a burning bush would be for the theologian.

An experiment not only demonstrates the presence or absence of an association between cause and effect and temporal order consistent with a causal relationship, but also provides the best possible demonstration that other possible causal factors have been eliminated. This confidence that other possible causes have been eliminated has been named internal validity (Campbell & Stanley, 1966; Cook & Campbell, 1979). The use of a control group eliminates many of the common threats to internal validity—such as the possibility that change in the experimental group occurred, not due to the independent variable (or treatment), but as a result of events in the surrounding environment or as a result of maturation of the group members during the period under study. Because control group members are equally subject to such extraneous factors and differ from the experimental group only in their nonexposure to the independent variable (or treatment), any difference between the two groups greater than chance must be due to the causal influence of the experimental variable.

Because they assign such high status to experiments, scientists tend to be very precise about what they mean by the term. Laymen are not so careful. We will often hear someone say something like, "I'm experimenting with a new brand of shampoo," or, "I just thought I would try filling up with gasohol as an experiment." It is not likely that many of these people are really conducting an experimental study.

Some scientists have struggled against this tide of misuse and have tried to teach the public the true meaning of the word *experiment.* Others have decided to abandon the term to common usage and develop a new term for scientific usage.

The term *clinical trial* has come to be widely used in biomedical research settings as one of the new terms for experiments. This term is used by the Society for Clinical Trials, a multidisciplinary group of professionals conducting research in biomedical areas. *Therapeutic trial* is sometimes used when the experiment is used to test a means of treatment or therapy. When the experiment tests a hypothesized means of prevention it is sometimes called a *prophylactic trial.*

The term *controlled trial* has also gained wide acceptance, especially in nonbiomedical areas. Perhaps the most widely accepted among epidemiologists is the term *randomized controlled trial*. This lengthy term is often simplified by using the acronym *RCT*, which we will use as a synonym for experimental study. It does not seem likely, however, that RCT will ever become muddied by common usage. Not many are likely to announce that they are "RCTing with a new brand of shampoo" or have "filled my tank with gasohol as a randomized controlled trial."

Elements of a Randomized Controlled Trial ⎯⎯⎯⎯⎯⎯

The term *randomized controlled trial* states the three basic elements of an RCT: (1) subjects are randomly assigned to two (or more) groups; (2) members of one group are used as controls and are not exposed to the independent variable; and (3) the impact of the independent variable is tried on the other group (or groups).

Random assignment has come to be increasingly recognized as the most essential element of the experimental method. Early examples of essentially experimental methods commonly do not use random assignment. It seems unlikely that Daniel just happened to randomly select himself for inclusion in the experimental group of his Biblical experiment on nutrition. In Lind's (1753) study of scurvy (which will be reported later in the chapter), the assignment of ten of the twelve subjects to treatments seems to have been largely a matter of chance but no attempt seems to have been made to assure randomness.

Today we recognize that the high internal validity of experimental results is due primarily to the fact that members of the experimental and control groups were not selected (or self-selected) on the basis of any characteristic but rather represent two 50 percent random samples from the study population. True random assignment means that every person in the study population had an equal chance of being assigned to either of the groups. This is not achieved by, for instance, assigning every second person to the control group. It is fairly well approximated by drawing names from a hat or goldfish bowl. True random assignment requires that the epidemiologist number all members of the study population and then use a table of random numbers to select the members for assignment to one group.

Once group assignments have been made, the members of the experimental group must be exposed to the variable under study—this may be a hypothesized cause of disease, a proposed means of prevention, or a possible cure. The control group must not be exposed to this variable. This raises the important issue of <u>fidelity of implementation</u>—was the treatment carried out as planned. It is important for the researcher to know if each member of the experimental group was, in fact, exposed to the variable under study and if each member of the control group was not, in fact, so exposed.

At the end of the experiment, the experimental group is compared to the control group. Any significant difference between the two may be presumed to be due to the action of the variable to which the experimental group was exposed and the control group was not. A statistical test of significance, such as chi-square or analysis of variance, will tell the researcher (at a preselected degree of certainty— usually 95 percent certainty or the .05 level) whether the differences found are probably true differences or are probably just random error due to chance. In other sciences this is usually the end of analysis for experimental results but in epidemiology a further level of analysis is possible.

Risk Calculation

In prospective studies of disease incidence it is possible to go beyond significance testing to tell us whether the differences between two groups are true differences. We can assess whether these differences are meaningful as well as real. This is possible through the calculation of relative and attributable risk.

<u>Relative risk</u> (risk ratio, rate ratio, or RR) is the ratio of the incidence in the group exposed to the causal variable under study (smokers, hypertensives, females, and so on) compared to the incidence in a reference group (nonsmokers, normotensives, males) not exposed to that variable. Where the variable under study is a preventive method, this is reversed. In that case it is the ratio of the incidence in the unexposed group compared to the incidence in the exposed group. It can best be thought of, perhaps, as the ratio of the incidence in the high-risk group to the incidence in the low-risk group. Thus, a relative <u>risk of 2.5</u> would mean that persons exposed to the factor were two-and-one-half times as likely to develop the disease as those not exposed to the factor.

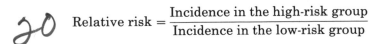

$$\text{Relative risk} = \frac{\text{Incidence in the high-risk group}}{\text{Incidence in the low-risk group}}$$

Attributable risk is the incidence in the high-risk group minus the incidence in the low-risk group. This represents the incidence in the high-risk group that can be attributed to the variable under study. That is, this is the rate of persons in the high-risk group who developed the disease who would not have done so had it not been for the variable under study. This gives us a measure of the amount of disease in the high-risk group that could be eliminated if that risk factor were eliminated.

Individually Randomized Controlled Trials

In the classic model of the randomized controlled trial, subjects are individually assigned to experimental and control groups. Although the degree of randomization varies, the following examples all illustrate individual assignment to groups.

An Early Experiment on the Treatment of Scurvy

Throughout human history various persons living on a diet deficient in fruits and fresh vegetables—such as sailors on long voyages—have suffered from the disease known as scurvy. Persons with scurvy first experience a loss of energy and pains in their legs, arms, and joints. As the condition progresses it produces symptoms of great weakness; spongy, bleeding gums; loosening of teeth; very bad breath; hemorrhages from the mucous membranes and under the skin; anemia; and painful hardening (known as brawny indurations) of areas in the muscles. The disease was frequently fatal.

In the mid-18th century, a number of theories were current about the cause and cure of scurvy. The British Naval physician James Lind (1753) performed a simple small scale experiment aboard HMS Salisbury in 1747 to test the rival treatments. He took aboard his ship 12 scurvy victims whose "cases were as similar as I could have them". The 12 men were housed together and fed the same diet. Six different treatments were tried on two men each. The selection of who was to receive each treatment was apparently a matter of chance, with the exception that two sailors, who seemed a bit sicker than the rest, were assigned to receive treatment with salt water—apparently the treatment in which Lind placed the most faith.

At the end of 6 days it was apparent that the two men whose treatment consisted of being given two oranges and one lemon to eat each day were showing the greatest improvement. One of the two, in fact, was fit to return to duty on the 6th day. The other 10 patients were likewise put on the citrus treatment and recovered. Based on these results, Lind recommended that all seamen should receive fruit daily to prevent scurvy. It took the British Navy only 50 years to adopt this recommendation, leading to the nickname "limey" for a British seaman.

An Experiment in Preventive Medicine for Heart Disease

The Multiple Risk Factor Intervention Trial (MRFIT) tested the effectiveness of multiple risk factor intervention conducted by physicians for men at high risk of ischemic heart disease. The study sample was identified by conducting screening programs in 20 U.S. communities over a 2-year period from 1973–1975. Over 370,000 men were examined and 12,866 subjects were identified who met the criteria of being currently free from symptoms of heart disease but being at high risk of heart disease due to cigarette smoking, high blood pressure, and elevated serum cholesterol.

Subjects were randomly assigned to either a special intervention (experimental) group or a usual care (control) group. The special intervention group was put on stepped-care drug treatment for their hypertension and was counseled on smoking cessation and dietary modification. The intervention began with a series of 10 weekly $1\frac{1}{2}$- to 2-hour intensive group sessions for the subjects and their wives. The purpose of these sessions was to provide information about the risk factors for heart disease and to initiate behavior change programs utilizing methods from behavior modification and group dynamics. Additional individual counseling was available for subjects who were not making progress toward their risk factor modification goals by the end of the initial 10 weeks.

Over an average followup period of 7 years, the mean risk factor levels for both groups were reduced. The experimental group, however, showed the greatest reductions in all three risk factors—smoking, blood pressure, and serum cholesterol.

The heart disease mortality rate for the experimental group was 17.9 deaths per 1,000 while that for the control group was 19.3 deaths per 1,000. This represents a statistically nonsignificant difference. Relative and attributable risk should not be calculated in such a case because the significance test indicates that the difference found is probably due to chance. Total mortality rates for the two groups were 41.2 deaths per 1,000 for the experimental group and 40.4 deaths per 1,000 for the control group. These rates also are not significantly different. The MRFIT results must, therefore, be interpreted as showing that the special intervention program had no more effect than ordinary care on the subsequent mortality of men at high risk for heart disease.

It should be clearly noted that the MRFIT only failed to support the value of the special intervention tested; it did not demonstrate that risk factor change was ineffective. Men in both groups who quit smoking experienced significantly lower heart disease mortality and total mortality than those men in either group who did not quit smoking. This evidence, of course, is not experimental in nature—quitting and not quitting were not randomly assigned so as to test their effects experimentally.

Community Trials

Often the independent variables that are of interest to epidemiologists are not of such a nature that they can be applied to individuals. We cannot, for instance, provide some individuals in a community with clean air to breathe while other randomly selected individuals breathe polluted air. To test the impact of community-wide variables we must conduct RCTs in which communities are randomly assigned to serve as experimental or control groups.

Community RCTs also increase the generalizability (or external validity) of research findings. Conducting trials in natural communities rather than laboratories or other contrived settings, which may be used in individually randomized RCTs, allows us to be more certain that the results of these studies will be applicable to the "real world." They do, however, present a number of statistical (Cornfield, 1978; Sherwin, 1978) and logistical (Farquhar, 1978) problems.

The Newburgh–Kingston Study

One of the classic community trials was the 10-year study of water fluoridation designed by David Ast (Ast & Schlesinger, 1956). Place studies had demonstrated that persons raised in areas where the water supply was naturally high in fluoride experienced about 60 percent less tooth decay (dental caries) than persons raised in areas with low fluoride levels in the water supply. The proposal to raise the fluoride level of public water supplies artificially had met with considerable controversy. Some argued that such a measure would not be effective, others that it would not be safe (Ast & Schlesinger, 1956). The U.S. Public Health Service and much of the dental profession had endorsed dentist-applied fluoride treatments in preference to water fluoridation. Ast was apparently among the opponents of fluoridation and expected his study to put an end to the idea of water fluoridation.

The two communities participating in this study were the cities of Newburgh and Kingston in New York. Located about 35 miles apart in the Hudson River valley, each city had a population of about 30,000 and similar ethnic and socioeconomic makeups. By the flip of a coin it was decided that Newburgh would serve as the experimental community and have its water supplemented with enough sodium fluoride to raise its fluoride level from 0.1 parts per million (ppm) to between 1.1 and 1.2 ppm. Kingston would serve as the control community with its fluoride level remaining unchanged at 0.1 ppm.

Prior to the fluoridation of the Newburgh water supply, extensive dental and medical examinations were conducted on 1,628 school children in Newburgh and 2,140 in Kingston. Periodic reexaminations were conducted throughout the 10-year study. Vital statistics regarding crude mortality, infant mortality, maternal mortality, cancer mortality, and so on were also monitored for both communities. Within a few years, the preliminary results had reversed Ast's position on the water fluoridation issue.

The baseline data had shown that there was no significant difference between the rates of dental caries in the two communities. Children aged 6–12 in Newburgh had a rate of 20.6 decayed, filled, or missing (DMF) teeth per 100 permanent teeth. In Kingston the rate was 20.2 DMF teeth per 100 permanent teeth. Over the 10 years of the study, the rate in Kingston remained essentially unchanged while that in Newburgh steadily declined to less than half the baseline rate.

Newburgh children aged 6–9, having drunk fluoridated water all their lives, had 57.9 percent less DMF teeth than children the same age in Kingston. Even 16-year-old Newburgh children, whose permanent teeth were already largely formed when water fluoridation began, showed 40.9 percent less DMF teeth than 16-year-olds drinking the unfluoridated water in Kingston.

In terms of relative risk, it can be said that the lack of water fluoridation caused the 6- to 9-year-old children in Kingston to suffer 2.37 times as much tooth decay as they would have if their water had been fluoridated. In terms of attributable risk, this amounts to about 10 decayed, filled, or missing teeth per 100 erupted permanent teeth.

The extensive medical examinations conducted on children in both communities failed to detect any effects of fluoridation. This included careful measures of growth and of bone density and maturation. Also included were tests of vision and hearing. Blood and urine analyses showed slightly more favorable results for children from Newburgh but no medically significant differences. Vital statistics revealed no effects on mortality in any age group or due to any cause. In brief, this and other similar experiments have shown that water fluoridation is both highly effective and quite safe.

The Stanford Three-Community Study

Another classic community RCT is the Stanford Heart Disease Prevention Project (Maccoby, Farquhar, Wood, & Alexander, 1977). This RCT tested the effectiveness of community health education as a means of reducing risk factors for heart disease and stroke.

Three communities in northern California served as the sites for the study. All three communities were within 60 miles of the researchers' base at Stanford University. Two of the communities, Watsonville and Gilroy, were served by the same television station but were separated by a small range of mountains, which minimized interaction despite their proximity. The third community, Tracy, was on the opposite side of Stanford and outside the range of the television station serving the other two communities. The communities were much alike in terms of population and economic factors.

Geography rather than randomization dictated that Tracy would be the control community, while Watsonville and Gilroy with their shared television station would be the targets of mass media messages about heart disease prevention. In addition to the use of television and radio messages, billboards, newspaper columns and advertisements, and mailed printed material in both experimental communities, two-thirds of a group of high-risk subjects in Watsonville were offered intensive counseling and followup services. The intensive services in Watsonville were offered to a randomly selected subgroup of high-risk individuals, which constitutes an embedded individual assignment RCT within the larger community study.

Pre- and postsurveys in the three communities showed 26 percent and 41 percent increases in knowledge of risk factor effects in the two experimental communities, with no increase in the control community. The group in Watsonville receiving the intensive intervention showed a 54 percent increase in knowledge.

Average levels of saturated fat consumption were reduced by approximately 25 percent in both experimental communities; serum cholesterol was reduced by 2–4 percent; cigarette smoking by 5–20 percent; and systolic blood pressure by 5–10 mm Hg. In Tracy, risk factors increased slightly.

Risk factor scores for a random sample of the population from each community showed an average decrease of 16 percent in Gilroy and 20 percent in Watsonville, with a 6 percent increase in Tracy. Looking only at high-risk individuals, those in Tracy showed a risk factor score reduction averaging less than 5 percent while those in Gilroy and Watsonville showed a reduction of 25 percent. The intensive intervention group in Watsonville reduced their risk factor scores an average of 30 percent.

A followup study known as the Stanford Five-Community Study is now underway, with two treatment and three control communities (Farquhar et al., 1985). In addition to improvements in the intervention methods and a sophisticated sampling design, this 7-year study will extend its outcome assessments to include incidence measures.

Natural Experiments

On rare occasions circumstances may arise in which a variable of possible causal importance is distributed in a population in a way that approximates random assignment. In these instances, differences between those exposed to the variable and those unexposed may be compared as though they were differences between an experimental group and a control group. These fortuitous occasions are known as "natural experiments."

A Natural Experiment on Cholera

John Snow (1855) was able to test his hypothesis that cholera was spread through fecal contamination of water in a natural experiment during the 1853 cholera epidemic. At this time a number of different companies competed selling water to the citizens of London. In the south of London many neighborhoods had their choice of water from either the Southwark & Vauxhall Company or the Lambeth Company. The pipes of the two companies passed together down all the streets of several south London districts. Some homeowners bought from one company, others from the other. Houses side-by-side might get their water from two different suppliers. In many cases, the choice had not been made by the current homeowner but by a previous owner.

Before 1852, it made little difference which water company served the house—both drew their water from highly contaminated parts of the Thames River. In 1852, however, the Lambeth Company moved their water works to a position upstream from the London sewers. From this time forward they provided water relatively free from fecal contamination while that from the Southwark & Vauxhall Company continued to be heavily contaminated.

During the 1853 cholera epidemic, Snow identified the deaths that occurred in houses served by each of these companies. Because he had no way of readily knowing the number of persons served by each company, he calculated rates based on deaths per 10,000 houses. He found that there were 315 deaths for every 10,000 houses served by Southwark & Vauxhall but only 37 deaths per 10,000 houses served by the Lambeth Company (Table 11.1).

From these results it can be seen that cholera deaths were 8.5 times more likely to occur in houses served by the Southwark & Vauxhall Company than those served by the Lambeth Company. In terms of attributable risk, 278 deaths occurred per 10,000 houses served by the Southwark & Vauxhall Company because they were served by that company instead of Lambeth.

The Vietnam Project

During the last years of the Vietnam War, a great deal of public concern was focused on drug use (especially heroin use) by U.S. servicemen in Vietnam. There was concern that such drug use was impairing their ability to fight. There was even greater concern about

TABLE 11.1   Cholera Mortality in Houses Served by Two Water Companies: London, 1854

Water Supplier	Number of Houses	Cholera Deaths	Deaths per 10,000 Houses
Southwark & Vauxhall Company	40,046	1,263	315
Lambeth Company	26,107	98	37

Source: Snow, J. (1855). *On cholera.* Cambridge, MA: Harvard University Press.

the impact on American society when drug addicted veterans returned from Vietnam. Lee Robins (1978) conducted an important study that addressed this problem.

A group of Vietnam veterans was identified, which consisted of a random sample of all Army enlisted males who returned from Vietnam in September of 1971. A control group was selected from the records of the Selective Service System; the members of this cohort were young men who were eligible for the draft but who held high lottery numbers and therefore had not been drafted. Members of the second group were individually matched with members of the veteran group on the basis of age, educational level, and place of residence at the time the veteran was inducted. Because lottery numbers were essentially random, these two groups—draftees with low lottery numbers and nondraftees with high lottery numbers—are essentially equivalent to randomly assigned groups. This is not quite true, of course, because the veteran group included a minority of volunteers who might be different from draftees.

Both groups were interviewed about 1 year and about 3 years after the veterans' return from Vietnam. Each veteran was interviewed concerning his drug use before induction, while in the Army, and since discharge. Nonveterans were asked about their drug use during the period matching those phases in the life of the veteran they were matched with.

As expected, the Vietnam veteran group showed much higher incidence rates for first use of marijuana and narcotics during their military service than did the nonveterans during the same peirod. However, an unexpected finding was that the veterans showed higher incidence rates than the nonveterans in all three time periods for marijuana, narcotics, barbiturates, and amphetamines. This was more true for the volunteers than for the draftees, but the draftees still showed higher incidence rates than their matched controls even before they were drafted.

Although the incidence rates for the two groups differed over all three time periods for all four drug groups, the curves were essentially the same for both groups for barbiturates and amphetamines—the veterans' incidence rates paralleling those of the nonveterans at a somewhat higher level. Both groups showed highest incidence during the second period and lowest during the third, indicating that the veterans had served in Vietnam during the period when they would have been at highest risk of drug use initiation in any case. For marijuana and narcotics the same pattern appears but the increase during the second period for the veterans is far greater than for the nonveterans. In summation, it appears that soldiers serving in Vietnam were at an age when they were most vulnerable to the initiation of illicit drug use and they therefore were greatly affected by the availability of marijuana, opium, and heroin in Vietnam and by the circumstances of combat service to initiate use of these drugs at an exceptionally high rate.

Recommended Reading

Bulpitt, C. J. (1983). *Randomized controlled clinical trials.* The Hague, Netherlands: Martinus Nijhoff Publishers.

Mattson, M. E., Curb, J. D., & McArdle, R. (1985). Participation in a clinical trial: The patients' point of view. *Controlled Clinical Trials, 6,* 156–167.

Pocock, S. (1984). *Clinical trials: A practical approach.* New York: John Wiley & Sons.

Symposium on CHD prevention trials: Design issues in testing lifestyle intervention. (1978). *American Journal of Epidemiology, 108,* 85–111.

CHAPTER 12

Cohort Studies

Often it is impractical or unethical to randomly assign a group of people to be exposed to an independent variable we wish to study. Given what we already know about the harmful effects of smoking, we cannot ask people to smoke so that we can study yet another possible ill-effect. Likewise, it would be unethical to randomly assign people to be exposed to radiation or toxic wastes. We can, however, study people who have already been exposed to toxic wastes, whose job exposes them to radiation, or who choose to smoke.

Such studies are much weaker than randomized controlled trials because we are less certain that other possible causes are being excluded. People who have been exposed to toxic wastes may have been exposed in the same fashion to other causal factors. Smokers may be different from nonsmokers in ways that have a causal impact on the disease we are studying (e.g., they may be more inclined to take risks or less concerned about their health). Despite these weaknesses, cohort studies are still of considerable value, providing far stronger evidence than the cross-sectional surveys of descriptive epidemiology.

The Cohort Method

The term *cohort* originally referred to a group of persons born the same year in the same place (nation, state, city, hospital, and so on).

Cohorts were studied primarily for mortality data. Studies of births in cohorts of women born the same year have also been used for quite some time as a way to study fertility. Today the term *birth cohort* is used for cohorts of this original type.

The term *cohort* is used today for any group that is followed up over time. Subjects are selected for inclusion in a cohort because of some current exposure to a possible cause. They are then followed up prospectively over time to measure the incidence of the disease under study. For this reason, cohort studies are also known as prospective studies and as incidence studies.

The Framingham Heart Study

One of the best known of all cohort studies is the Framingham Heart Study. This study was initiated in 1948 by the U.S. Public Health Service and researchers at the Harvard School of Public Health to study a variety of possible risk factors for heart disease. The town of Framingham in Massachusetts (population 28,000) was chosen as the site of the study because of its relatively stable population, availability of a local community hospital, proximity to Boston and Harvard, and cooperation in a previous community study. The study was originally planned as a 20-year followup but has now been underway almost twice that long.

A list of all local residents was developed as a sampling frame for random selection. Families were listed together within each precinct. Two out of every three families (6,507 persons) were invited to participate. Of these, 4,469 persons agreed to participate. Because this was less than the researchers' goal of 5,000 participants, a group of 740 volunteers was added to make a total of 5,209 subjects.

All of these subjects were then given a physical examination that included measures of blood pressure and serum cholesterol. At this stage, 82 subjects were found to have symptoms indicative of previously undiagnosed heart disease and were removed from the sample, leaving a total of 5,127. These persons could be subdivided into subcohorts based on such characteristics as smokers versus nonsmokers or hypertensives versus normotensives. The cohort has been offered a relatively comprehensive physical examination every 2 years. This not only provides some outcome data but allows reassignment to subcohorts as conditions change and has allowed the addition of some new measurements of interest that were not part of the original study design.

Much of our current knowledge of risk factors for heart disease either came out of this study or was confirmed by the study. The findings with regard to the role of serum cholesterol in heart disease were particularly important. In males aged 30–49, for instance, the risk of heart disease in those with serum cholesterol levels greater than 250 mg% is 4.1 times that of men with cholesterol levels below 190 mg%.

The existence of this long-standing cohort, on which numerous variables have been recorded, has permitted numerous studies that were not included in the original plan. For instance, although this cohort was created to study heart disease, the causes of all deaths in the cohort have been recorded, allowing studies of mortality of any type and not just heart disease mortality. For example, mortality due to all causes has been studied in relationship to alcohol consumption. Gordon and Kannel (1984) found that there is no association between drinking and subsequent mortality in women. Among men, although increased alcohol consumption is associated with increased mortality due to cirrhosis of the liver and cancer (especially stomach cancer), non-drinkers suffer higher mortality than drinkers, even the heaviest drinkers. Although contrary to many peoples' expectations, these findings are consistent with those from other cohort studies of drinking and mortality.

Coffee Consumption and Cancer Mortality

In 1966, a prospective study of 26,020 male life insurance policy-holders was initiated. A dietary frequency-of-use survey was mailed to this population and was completed and returned by 17,818 men, who became the cohort under study. Cancer mortality among heavy coffee users was compared to all other subjects. The hypothesized relationship between heavy coffee drinking and pancreatic cancer was not found. No positive relationships were found between coffee consumption and any form of cancer except lung cancer. Even after controlling for age, urban/rural residence, and cigarette use, the relative risk of death due to lung cancer was 7.33 times as great for heavy coffee drinkers. This compares to a relative risk of 9.6 for cigarette smokers, controlling for the influence of age, urban/rural residence, and coffee consumption. Persons who drink five or more cups of coffee per day and smoke a pack or more of cigarettes per day are 40.37 times more likely to die of lung cancer.

Historical Cohorts ───────────────────────────────────

The major disadvantage of cohort studies is the amount of time it takes to complete them. We often need answers now that can only be provided by a 20-year prospective study. Sometimes we can obtain the answers sooner by way of a historical cohort study. The opportunity to conduct such a study is present when we can find some record that allows us to assign some population to groups based on their exposure to a possible cause at some time in the past and to follow those people until the present time, keeping track of the incidence of the disease under study.

Radiation and Mortality

The end of World War II thrust us into the Atomic Age with little idea of what the health consequences of radiation might be. Although it was obvious that large doses of radiation can be lethal, the cumulative effects of smaller doses were unknown. Unfortunately, to study this question through standard cohort or experimental methods would have required decades and the answers then might come too late.

Seltser and Sartwell (1965) devised a historical cohort study to assess the possible hazards of small doses of radiation. They studied mortality among members of three professional organizations. The three organizations were the Radiologic Society of North America (founded in 1915), the American College of Physicians (founded in 1915), and the American Academy of Ophthalmology and Otolaryngology (founded in 1921). Members were studied from the time they joined their professional organization until 1958.

As radiologists, the first group had substantial exposure daily to radiation, especially during this period when modern precautions were not taken. The second group, being composed of internists, was likely in those days to have quite a bit of x-ray exposure but far less than the radiologists. The third group, being eye, ear, nose, and throat (ENT) specialists, made little if any use of x-rays and thus served as a low-risk cohort.

Mortality was studied for the periods 1935–1944, 1945–1954, and 1955–1958. In all three periods, mortality rates were highest for the radiologists and lowest for the ENT specialists. Radiologists, for instance, showed a mortality due to leukemia that was 2.5 times as great as that of the ENT specialists. Radiation exposure was clearly associated with greater mortality due to cancer, heart disease, kidney disease, and all causes combined. The precautions taken by modern radiologists owe much to this study.

Recommended Reading

Cook, N. R., & Ware, J. H. (1983). Design and analysis methods for longitudinal research. *Annual Review of Public Health, 4,* 1–23.

Dawber, T. R., Kannel, W. B., & Lyell, L. P. (1963). An approach to longitudinal studies in a community: The Framingham Study. *Annals of the New York Academy of Sciences, 107,* 593–599.

Kandel, D. B. (Ed.). (1978). *Longitudinal research on drug use: Empirical findings and methodological issues.* New York: John Wiley & Sons.

Stallones, R. A. (1966). Prospective epidemiologic studies of cerebrovascular disease. In *Cerebrovascular disease epidemiology: A workshop* (Public Health Monograph No. 76). Washington, DC: U.S. Government Printing Office.

CHAPTER 13

Case-Control Studies

The index case, the one from which an investigation begins, was a 15-year-old girl who was admitted to Children's Hospital in Denver with a 105.6-degree fever. She was clinically described as being "confused," "aggressive," and in a state of shock with a systolic blood pressure of 66. A red rash covered her body. She suffered periods of vomiting and diarrhea.

Treated with a battery of nonspecific therapies, she seemed on the way to recovery when, on the third day of her hospitalization, skin peeled from the soles of her feet and from her abdomen. Gangrene developed in two toes of her left foot, requiring their amputation. After a week in the hospital, she was released, well on the road to recovery but still undiagnosed.

Her physician, Dr. James Todd, identified six more cases of the same mysterious condition in three boys and three more girls, aged 8–17. All had shown symptoms of rash, lowered blood pressure, fever, gastrointestinal problems, and mental confusion. One of the cases had been fatal. The other five had survived but had undergone a period of "fine desquamation"—shedding of skin—from their palms and soles during the recovery period.

Tests for a number of suspected agents proved negative. The tests did identify in all seven patients the presence of the common bacterium *Staphylococcus aureus*. This bacteria is commonly found on the skin and in the nose and throat of healthy persons, but when it gets beneath the surface of the skin it can cause an assortment of infectious conditions including boils, carbuncles, and the childhood disease of impetigo.

S. aureus is also the agent responsible for most wound infections—the agent Lister had hypothesized might live harmlessly on the skin surface but would cause postsurgical sepsis when it entered the intima of the body (see Chapter 1). It can also produce serious infections of the respiratory, gastrointestinal, and urinary tracts. In one fairly rare childhood condition, known as *Ritter's disease*, infection of the epidermis results in a toxic byproduct that causes a rash, fever, superficial blisters, and desquamation.

Dr. Todd named this severe new condition *toxic shock syndrome* (or TSS). Being a pediatrician, he and his colleagues had seen cases only in children. Therefore, they described toxic shock syndrome as a disease of older children—a classic example of the incompleteness of the clinical picture. Reports of cases from Wisconsin and Minnesota soon established that TSS was not a disease of children only.

With the growing number of reports, the Centers for Disease Control (CDC) began to investigate TSS. Their first report on TSS identified 55 cases, 52 of whom were women, almost all of whom reported that the onset of the illness followed the start of their menstrual period. The virulence of the disease was high, with 10–15 percent of the cases being fatal.

Soon afterward, CDC researchers conducted a quick telephone survey in which they contacted 52 women who had suffered toxic shock syndrome and an equal number of their friends who had not. The women were questioned about their marital status, frequency of sexual intercourse, intercourse during menstruation, birth control practices, history of herpes or other vaginal infections, use of douches or sprays during menstruation, and use of tampons and sanitary napkins. Tabulations revealed that TSS cases were significantly more likely than noncases to use tampons, especially continual use. No differences were found on any of the other variables.

In a subsequent study, tampon usage patterns of 50 women who had come down with TSS during the preceding 2 months were compared to 150 healthy women. Again, tampon usage was shown to be highly associated with TSS. Furthermore, one brand of tampon, the RELY brand, was shown to have been used by an exceptionally large proportion of the cases.

It was eventually demonstrated that the incidence of TSS among women who did not use tampons was less than one per 100,000, while the incidence among tampon users was six cases per 100,000. The relative risk associated with tampon use was thus more than six. Of the first 299 reported cases of TSS, 71 percent were users of RELY tampons. As a result of the CDC's findings, the manufacturers of RELY tampons removed their product from the market. The exact mechanism by which tampons cause TSS remains unknown, as do the reasons why RELY tampons were more dangerous than other brands.

The Case-Control Method

The history given above of the investigation of toxic shock syndrome is a good illustration of the case-control method. In a case-control study, a group of persons who have experienced the disease under study are compared to an otherwise similar group who have not had the disease. The past histories of both groups are examined for the presence of possible causes.

This is the precise opposite of a cohort study, in which persons are assigned to groups in the present based on presence or absence of a hypothesized cause and are then followed into the future to measure the incidence of disease. In the case-control study, persons are assigned to groups based on presence or absence of the disease and are then traced back into the past to measure the frequency of hypothesized causes.

Case-control studies are an outgrowth of the ages-old medical practice of case studies. Physicians have long published detailed reports of single cases or groups of cases that they feel are representative of a new or understudied disease or health condition. Such case studies commonly have included a retrospective examination of possible causal events in the patients' past histories. The use of a formal control group to improve the ability to identify actual causal factors is a fairly recent development. With this addition, the frequently valueless case study was converted into a useful analytic tool.

The major problem in using this tool, however, has been the difficulty of identifying an appropriate control group. One popular strategy, as in the telephone study of TSS reported above, is to use the best friends of cases; a persons's best friend is apt to be very much like him or her in many ways. A similar strategy is to use the coworkers of cases, or their roommates or siblings. Another strategy is to use patients at the same hospital or clinic who are suffering from unrelated conditions. In a case-control study of child abuse, Hawkins and Duncan (1985a) used as controls persons who had been reported as child-abuse suspects but who had been cleared of the charges in comparison to substantiated cases reported to the same agency. A sample from the general population is sometimes used as a control group.

The Odds Ratio in Case-Control Studies

It is not possible to calculate relative or attributable risk from case-control studies. These calculations are based on comparing the incidence rates of two groups in a cohort or experimental study. In a case-control study, the incidence rate in one group—the cases—is always 100 percent while the incidence rate among the controls is always 0 percent.

However, it is possible to estimate relative risk from a case-control study. This estimate is known as the odds ratio or relative odds. Traditionally, the calculation of this statistic is taught by instructing the learner to put the results in a table format, as shown in Figure 13.1.

Each cell in the table is represented by a letter, *A* through *D*. Relative odds can then be calculated by substituting each cell value for the corresponding letter in the following formula:

$$\text{Relative odds} = \frac{A \times D}{B \times C}$$

For those who do not wish to trust their memorization of a precise table set-up, it may be more useful to learn the odds ratio by the following formula:

$$\text{Relative odds} = \frac{AB}{aB} \Big/ \frac{Ab}{ab} = \frac{AB \times ab}{aB \times Ab}$$

	Case	Control
Factor present	A	B
Factor absent	C	D

Figure 13.1   Format of Table for Calculation of Relative Odds.

given that $AB =$ factor present and disease present, $Ab =$ factor present and disease absent, $aB =$ factor absent and disease present, and $ab =$ factor absent and disease absent.

Utilizing this formula, you can see that we are (1) multiplying the number of cases who were exposed to the factor times the number of controls who were not, and (2) dividing this sum by the sum of the number of cases that were not exposed to the factor times the number of controls who were. For a mathematical discussion of these and alternate procedures, see Kahn (1983).

As an illustration, we might take the findings of Zunzunegui, King, Coria, and Charlet (1986) regarding the number of sexual partners of husbands of women with cervical cancer. Of 78 husbands of women with cervical cancer, 48 (62 percent) reported having had 20 or more sexual partners. Of the 78 husbands of matched controls, only 22 (27 percent) reported having had 20 or more sexual partners. This may be formatted as shown in Figure 13.2. Relative odds can then be calculated, as follows:

$$\frac{A \times D}{B \times C} = \frac{48 \times 56}{22 \times 30} = \frac{2688}{660} = 4.07$$

or

$$\frac{AB}{aB} \bigg/ \frac{Ab}{ab} = \frac{48}{30} \bigg/ \frac{22}{56} = \frac{48 \times 56}{30 \times 22} = \frac{2688}{660} = 4.07$$

	Husbands of cases	Husbands of controls
Less than 20 sexual partners	16 (A)	51 (B)
20 or more sexual partners	62 (C)	27 (D)

Figure 13.2   Format of Table for Calculation of Relative Odds.

In other words, we would estimate from these data that women whose husbands have 20 or more sexual partners are four times as likely to develop cervical cancer as are women whose husbands have fewer sex partners. This is consistent with the hypothesis that cervical cancer has a viral agent that is spread as a venereal infection.

Alcohol and Sudden Cardiac Death

There is a tendency among health professionals to view alcohol only in terms of alcohol abuse and the possible harm done to the individual drinking alcohol. Actually, however, there is a growing body of evidence regarding the health benefits of drinking. Numerous studies have shown that moderate drinking (usually defined as no more than two drinks per day but sometimes defined as no more than four per day) is associated with greater longevity. Furthermore, nondrinkers show higher mortality than heavy drinkers. Evidence has also accumulated suggesting that moderate alcohol consumption is protective against heart disease.

Siscovick, Weiss, and Fox (1986) undertook a case-control study to assess the role of alcohol drinking in relation to sudden cardiac death. They compared 152 cases between the ages of 25 and 72 and without previous history of heart disease, who had died of a sudden primary cardiac arrest. Controls were 152 demographically similar residents of the same county. The spouses of both the cases and the controls were interviewed about the case's (or control's) average alcohol consumption.

After adjustment to eliminate the influence of smoking, hypertension, and physical activity, it was found that alcohol consumption was apparently associated with lower rates of sudden cardiac death. Compared to nondrinkers, the odds ratio for light drinkers (less than one drink per day) was 0.7. For moderate drinkers (1–3 drinks per day) the odds ratio was 0.5. In other words, this study shows that moderate drinkers have about half the chance of sudden cardiac death that nondrinkers have.

This study illustrates one of the advantages of a case-control study. It can be used to study relatively rare events such as sudden cardiac death. Had this been examined in a prospective study comparing drinkers to nondrinkers, both groups would have to have been very large due to the low incidence of sudden cardiac death.

Recommended Readings ————————————————————

Breslow, N. (1982). Design and analysis of case-control studies. *Annual Review of Public Health, 3,* 29–54.

Cornfield, J., & Haenzel, W. (1960). Some aspects of retrospective studies. *Journal of Chronic Disease, 11,* 523–525.

Kahn, H. A. (1983). Relative risk and odds ratio. In *An introduction to epidemiologic methods.* New York: Oxford University Press.

Schlesselman, J. J. (1982). *Case-control studies: Design, conduct, analysis.* New York: Oxford University Press.

CHAPTER 14

Investigations of Epidemics and Outbreaks

Victoria C. Markellis, M.D., M.P.H.
Associate Professor of Health Science
State University of New York
Brockport, NY

In the not too distant past, the investigation of epidemics and outbreaks was limited only to communicable diseases. Today, investigation of the infectious diseases still poses an urgent, active part of epidemiology. With the propagation of conditions that are not "infectious" but still fit into the criteria of the epidemiologic triangle, the investigation of epidemics has taken on further interesting and exciting dimensions. Investigators in other disciplines and fields have recognized the value of the epidemiological model, and its methods have been sought and accepted.

Even though new methods have been adopted and adapted from disciplines such as sociology, biology, demography, and others, and the scope of epidemiology has increased and entered fields such as management and story telling, the epidemiologist must not be wrongfully persuaded that there necessarily must be different ways to investigate and analyze the communicable and the noncommunicable diseases and conditions (Lilienfeld, 1973). Both groups are studied by the same methods, and the same reasoning processes should be applied.

Understanding Methods

Because epidemiology and its methods have been sought and accepted by a variety of disciplines, it is even more important that the methods for investigation of epidemics and/or outbreaks be appropriately understood and followed to attain one's goal. An investigation is a painstaking, exacting exercise by the epidemiologic detective and the investigating team, a step-by-step operation in puzzle solving. *Nothing must be left to chance* in order to fulfill the purpose of the study, which is to prevent any continuance of the epidemic or the recurrence of the condition, regardless of the cause. The investigator must master a methodical procedure if he or she is to reach a correct and successful answer.

The procedure is not one that gives a "quick answer." An investigation takes many hours, sometimes days or many weeks, of difficult, meticulous work. This work may be pursued by one person or by a team of persons, depending on the size of the problem and the size and location of the organization undertaking the investigation. The steps toward solving the "puzzle" sometin. 's fall into an orderly pattern. At other times, many individuals may be involved in a number of lesser investigations that may be brought together to the final analysis of finding the cause and to the developing of preventive measures.

Establishing the Correct Diagnosis

The first step, regardless of how the suspected case is reported or discovered, is to establish a correct diagnosis. A suspected case is one that has alerted a physician, public health nurse, hospital, or laboratory personnel that an individual has symptoms that may resemble a condition to be investigated. This, therefore, causes the investigator to further examine, test, and probe until a suspected case is confirmed as a case, or is denied and declared nonexistent.

A case of a disease or condition cannot be so labeled until signs and symptoms of the victim or host are analyzed and verified by a qualified person—usually a physician—and the "condition" is further confirmed by qualified laboratory findings. Under no other condition should an epidemiological investigator accept the report as a case. Until the correct diagnosis and verification of the disease or condition at hand is made, there can be no justified preventive measures taken. Assumption should not be part of the investigating epidemiologist's lexicon. An example of incorrect procedure is the following fictional case.

An investigator "assumes" that a case of a jaundiced cook in a large eating establishment is a case of infectious hepatitis when, in fact, the individual has a gallstone lodged in the common bile duct. With such skimpy evidence, an overzealous investigating public health team prematurely closes the restaurant; publicizes erroneous information in newspapers and newsletters, and on radio and television; sets up an expensive preventive gamma globulin immunizations program for persons exposed to food prepared by the cook; and as a result causes panic in the community. The team has carried out time consuming, expensive public health procedures. It has also caused unnecessary panic, caused the restaurant owner embarrassment and monetary loss, and could have caused a lawsuit against the health department. These problems could have been avoided if the team had established the correct diagnosis of the condition at hand.

Establishing the Existence of an Epidemic _____

Once the proper diagnosis has been made and verified, the investigating team must obtain a complete and proper history on the case or cases. It is of vital importance to obtain a thorough tabulation of contacts of the cases. Of further importance are (1) the knowledge of the disease or condition at hand, the symptoms, incubation and generation times, and length of communicability; and (2) the modes of transmission—so that proper laboratory samples are obtained and crucial testing may be done.

At all times during the investigation the team must keep uppermost in the study, the normal endemic occurrence in the community of the condition being examined. A well functioning health department should be the best source for information regarding the presence or absence of a disease in a community. The number of cases of a specific disease or infectious agent that is habitually present within a certain geographic area is called the *endemic occurrence*. This occurrence is normally expected in the community at all times; the "normal expected presence" varies for different geographic areas for different diseases. For instance, in the 1940s it was estimated that about 80 countries reported smallpox and that a majority of the world's population lived in smallpox-endemic areas, yet the United States had no cases reported (Hanlon & Pickett, 1979).

However, when the normal expected presence is exceeded an epidemic exists. The term *epidemic* may encompass any kind of disease, communicable or noncommunicable, or any type of injury or condition. ⑥

An epidemic must be investigated with the basic descriptive factors in mind: person, place, and time. Again, by being knowledgeable about the disease or condition, the investigator may save endless hours of unfounded work and research by knowing the proper population to investigate. An epidemic of chickenpox, measles, or diphtheria most likely would be present in a child population, whereas a study of hypertension cases or degenerative types of arthritis most likely would be in an elderly population. Limitation of an epidemic may be to one specific geographic area, such as a city, village, county, or state, or it may be widespread and become worldwide, as do yearly influenza epidemics and pandemics. ⑦

Time experience of an epidemic may also vary. Influenza strikes worldwide in the late fall and early winter months. Chickenpox, on the other hand, occurs yearly in the United States on a cyclic course in the months January to April. Further, the duration of individual communicable diseases may vary widely. A case of staphylococcus food "poisoning" caused by staphylococcal enterotoxin may last a few hours to a few days. The onset of an epidemic of this condition usually is explosive, lasts for a short time, and has a common source. Influenza, on the other hand, may last for a period of 2–3 weeks in an individual but the epidemic may last in the community from a few weeks through many months as various parts of the world population become affected. Injury epidemics, depending on the type and cause, may last from a few weeks to many years or until conditions are corrected.

The epidemiological detective must be aware of incidence of a disease, present and past, so that he or she may determine the comparison of the present experience to that of the past. The epidemiologist must further be able to (1) determine the rate at which people at risk without the disease are developing the disease within a specified period of time; and (2) measure the amount of a disease existing at a given point in time—the *prevalence*. ⑧

The collection of samples and specimens is of significant importance. Many suspected diagnoses have been lost or unconfirmed because of loss of a sample. Incorrect sampling techniques, lack of knowledge by the investigator of proper specimens collection, and improper time of sampling will allow suspected cases to remain in that category. ⑨

Epidemiological Study of the Epidemic _____

This portion of the study is the ['shoe leather]' portion of epidemiology. One by one cases and contacts of the condition are sought out and identified, and careful data identifying any relevant pieces of information are collected. Name or identifying number, age, sex, race, address, geographic area, type of life style, religion, occupation, associations to which the individual belongs, social activities, family relations, and so on must be gathered. Depending on the disease or condition involved, it may be necessary to gather many other variables.

A successful epidemiological investigator must possess the following characteristics: curiosity, the love of puzzle solving, the ability to gather information meticulously, the ability to record and separate this information in an orderly manner, a basic suspiciousness, a tremendous amount of energy, an unbelievable tenacity, an understanding of human psychology, knowledge of diseases, and a tremendous amount of patience. This detective must also be able to tabulate data honestly and to analyze data objectively. His or her basic statistical knowledge must be impeccable.

Description and characterization of the epidemic is vital to its proper study and analysis. Following the orderly gathering of data (individual data forms for each case), each case must be tabulated in an easily understood manner. A table form is probably the most legible form of grouping information. Table 14.1 is a simple example of tabulation.

In the simple fictitious example in Table 14.1, the analyst can see that the cases of illness occurred in the male Cub Scouts who attended a jamboree on June 15 and became ill on June 17 or 18. The details of the individual's illness may be studied from his individual symptom and data sheet, and numerous other tables may be constructed from the information.

An epidemic curve that gives an investigator a "picture" of the time of illness and frequency of cases should be made. By placing cases on an epidemic curve by onset of diseases (Figure 14.1), the investigator can clearly visualize when cases had their true onset of symptoms, classify the condition at hand, and determine whether the outbreak may be a possible common source or a propagated or progressive epidemic.

By closer studying times of eating at the jamboree in Figure 14.1, another epidemic curve can be constructed by hours of food consumption and hours of symptom onset.

The investigator must be knowledgeable about specifying disease differences, and a thorough and patient questioner and listener. Onset

TABLE 14.1

Name or Identifying Number of Cases	Age	Sex	Race	Illness	No Illness	Cub Scout Member	Attended Jamboree June 15	Date of Illness
Graves, Yvon	7	M	W	x		x	x	June 18 (3)
Smith, Mary	5	F	B		x	x		
Jones, Joseph	9	M	B	x		x	x	June 17 (1)
Brown, Jo	8	F	W		x	x		
Green, Marion	9	M	W	x		x	x	June 18 (4)
White, Marian	8	F	B		x	x		
Gray, Lavel	9	M	Ind.	x		x	x	June 17 (2)
Broad, Loren	9	M	W	x		x	x	June 18 (5)

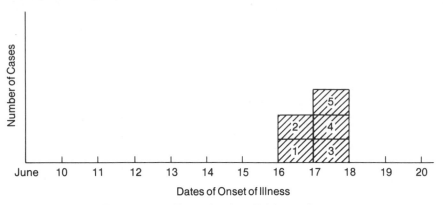

Figure 14.1 Example of an Epidemic Curve.

of symptoms must be clearly obtained from the victims—it is extremely important to know when each individual first became ill. The question that should be given priority is: "When did this person first not feel his normal self?" The first difference should be noted, *not* what the investigator thinks the first difference should be. The investigator should *not* implant in the patient's mind what he or she, the investigator, wants to hear. For instance, a foodborne illness victim may first experience "nausea" or salivation or a "queasy feeling." This is the onset of illness for that particular individual. The investigator, however, may ask, "When did you get diarrhea?," a symptom that may come later than the onset but one that the investigator may only associate with intestinal infection—he or she may not know that this particular symptom may have an onset in this particular disease many hours after the onset. It is, therefore, of utmost importance that the investigator is fully trained, experienced, and knowledgeable about history taking, symptomatology, and disease concepts.

The maintenance of a spot map or pin map is of utmost value. Location of residence of cases in a community may be helpful in pinpointing location of cause—such as a contaminated water supply or as in the past, pre- milk pasteurization days, when a contaminated milk source supplied milk to a certain population on a particular route. In other cases, a spot map may show no residence proximity of cases but may help the analyst understand that the contaminations happened in a common source area, such as at a social, school, or business event. The investigators are saved hours of potentially wasted time in searching for irrelevant cases. By probing meticulously into time, place, and person, the investigator can narrow the areas to be investigated. If cases are children, there may be no need to seek out older citizens for investigation. If the cases attended one school function at the food outlet in that school, hours of valuable time are saved by concentrating on that population.

The characteristic incubation period of the disease, if it is a communicable disease, may further help to seek out an activity at the beginning of that time that may be relevant to the cases. Methodically, the location of the victim can be established when disease could have been acquired.

Therefore, knowledge of incubation periods of diseases is one of the *14* most important features in epidemiological study of communicable diseases. The incubation period is that period of time from the host's exposure to the agent to the time of onset of illness. It is imperative that the investigator have the knowledge of the variety of incubation periods of diseases.

Communicable diseases are easily depicted by their incubation times. *15* When investigating chronic diseases, however, much difficulty enters the picture. When the exposure to a carcinogenic factor occurred many years before the malignancy becomes evident in the patient, it will often be unrecognized or forgotten.

After the careful construction of an epidemic curve with proper identification of onset times of illness, the study team must determine that a position must be set forth. The team must decide whether this *16* epidemic appears to be a common source epidemic or one that is being spread from individual to individual. A common source epidemic is one in which the victims were exposed to an agent at one point in time and, usually, at the same place. The epidemic curve in a common source epidemic clusters about the median incubation time of that disease. The investigators can concentrate on the events that occurred about that time.

17 A propagated epidemic is one in which the agent is transmitted, directly or indirectly, from one susceptible host to another. In plotting an epidemic curve of a propagated epidemic, one finds that cases continue to appear beyond one incubation period, which is much different from the concentrated number of cases in the common source epidemic.

To determine causative factors in an epidemic, data collected must be carefully analyzed. Those individuals exposed to possible sources of a suspected agent are compared to persons not exposed. The attack rate or *18* incidence is compared in the two groups. If those persons who were exposed to the possible source display a much higher rate than those not exposed, a differential is determined and the probability of the source is narrowed. Table 14.2 presents an imaginary foodborne illness case.

TABLE 14.2 Attack Rates of Illness According to Food Histories in an Epidemic of "Food Poisoning"

Food Items Served	Persons Who Ate Specified Food				Persons Who Did Not Eat Specified Food				Difference in Attack Rate
	Illness Cases	No Illness Cases	Total	Illness Percent	Illness Cases	No Illness Cases	Total	Illness Percent	
Tossed salad with dressing	36	12	48	75%	40	14	54	74%	+1.0%
Green peas with butter sauce	48	20	68	70.5%	28	6	34	82.3%	−11.8%
Chicken a la King	74	17	91	81.3%	2	9	11	18.2%	+63.1%
Buttered biscuits	46	12	58	79.1%	30	14	44	68.2%	+10.9%
Chocolate mousse	62	22	84	73.8%	14	4	18	77.8%	+4.0%
Milk	60	16	76	78.9%	16	10	26	61.5%	+17.4%

Note the comparisons of individuals who ate the food and became ill with those who did not but became ill. An attack rate can also be called *percent ill.* In a foodborne outbreak, that food which has the highest difference between attack rates of persons eating food (exposed) and persons not eating food (not exposed) is usually the food containing the causative agent.

Food-specific attack rate is determined by the following formula:

$$\text{Food-specific attack rate} = \frac{\text{Number of persons eating specific food and becoming ill}}{\text{Total number of persons eating specific food}}$$

In Table 14.2, the number of persons who ate each food and became ill was calculated and the total number of persons eating the food was recorded. Therefore, the food-specific attack rate for each food eaten with subsequent illness would be compared to those who were ill but did not eat the food. The difference between these two rates is calculated. By proceeding through the entire food list and comparing differentials of attack rates, the analysis shows that symptoms of the illness were caused by an agent that was in the vehicle—Chicken a la King.

By investigating the suspect food—source of ingredients, handling techniques, storage practices, mode of preparation, serving, personnel background, and food preparation habits—the public health sanitarian, nurse, physician, and epidemiologist can target the exact source and "modus operandi" of the agent.

The basic purpose of epidemiological investigation then can be called into action—the prevention of the condition. Proper means can be brought to bear so that the source of contamination can be found and eliminated, unsanitary personnel habits can be corrected, or food preparation habits can be altered.

Reporting the Epidemic

In many fields, workers are required to write, present, publicize, or file a report on their job activities. A report in the field of epidemiology is not only "part of the job" but it becomes a very important part of the investigation or study as well. Depending on the cause of an epidemic, the report may be an anxiously awaited for and often a critical part of the investigation. The report may be the last act of the team or a beginning of a new investigation; it may form a new hypothesis or may set forth a direction for curtailing one epidemic and preventing others.

The form of the report will vary depending on the requirements of an agency, company, or any other employer of the team of investigators. Nevertheless, the materials to be included in the report will be those data mentioned earlier and, of course, the report will be only as good as the data and details collected, and the ability, insight, and clarity of thinking of the reporter.

Depending on the type of epidemic and the agent involved, the report may take on a variety of forms. The form or forms used will depend on the basic purpose of the report and to whom the report will be submitted. The basic premise is that the report will inform its audience but the type of audience and the setting of the report-giving will determine the form of the report.

Content

The investigator or team must know at early stages of the investigation or study what will constitute the report. The data, needless to say, must be accurate, but the content to be handled helps to organize the reporter's material. He or she must keep in mind the material to be gathered step-by-step, the transition that the report must take, and the type of audience.

The audience's diverse needs for facts, findings, and evidence that are vital and complex must always be kept in mind. What an investigator reports to a public health department director or to a board of health must necessarily be much different than a report given to a newspaper for the public consumption, in order to alleviate possible panic. The basic information and facts should not differ but the way in which they are presented should.

Format

Depending on where the report will be submitted, it may take on a variety of forms. The presentation of an epidemiological report may be an internal report prepared for an organization or agency usually consisting of scientific, health related professionals, or it may be external covering a variety of audiences with a variety of needs and understandings.

Internally, the report may be written to include required facts, figures, and evaluations. The investigator may find it necessary to present materials in office memos or bulletins to fellow epidemiologists, or to a variety of agency departments. A required system report may have to be filed or sent to a branch agency.

Externally, the epidemiologist may be required to fill mandated state or federal agency report forms, with conclusions and recommendations. Press releases become vital parts of epidemic reporting. What and how it is included in these reports may alleviate fear and panic in the community. An oral report of epidemiological findings may have to be made as the epidemic progresses or at the conclusion of the investigation. Oral reports may be presented to committees or investigating team member groups, as one-on-one communication, or to a professional staff meeting of the agency. Externally, the investigator may be badgered by TV or radio reporters for oral reports of the epidemic. As a result he may or she may participate in newspaper interviews or conduct speeches to groups in the community.

On occasion, it may be more efficient, informative, and educational to use a graphic format both internally and externally to present the epidemiological report. Flip charts, overhead projections, slides, or films may better display comparative facts, findings, rates, and other pertinent information regarding the epidemic than any other form of reporting. The epidemiologist, therefore, must be able to compile and present pertinent material clearly, accurately, and professionally.

Function and Responsibilities of the Epidemic Control Epidemiologist

The function of the infection control epidemiologist is one of the most exciting, interesting, and stimulating occupations. The responsibilities of surveillance, studying epidemics, and implementing effective control measures are exercises for individuals who are energetic, curious, and have a desire to "set things right."

The monitoring or surveillance activity that the epidemiologist undertakes is one that involves a constant overseeing of the community. He or she is a policeman on the move, a detective who is always watching for clues. The school, the hospital, the industry, the small store, the large company, and many other community organizations may hold the causative agent or the solution to a difficult puzzle. The information that the epidemiologist holds may be the foundation for solving serious problems.

TABLE 14.3 Selected Foodborne Illnesses (Etiological Agents, Sources, Symptoms, and Methods of Prevention)

Disease and Etiological Agent	Source	Symptoms	Methods of Prevention
Staphylococcal foodborne illness *Agent:* Staphylococcal enterotoxin produced by *Staphylococcus aureus* bacteria.	Bacteria found on human skin and in throat flora. Toxin produced when contaminated food left out at room temperature. May be on meats, poultry, egg products, potato and macaroni salads, cream-filled desserts.	*Symptoms:* Severe diarrhea, vomiting, abdominal cramps, prostration. *Onset:* 1–8 hrs. after eating. Rarely fatal.	• Education of food personnel. • Sanitary food-handling practices. • Proper and prompt refrigeration of foods.
Salmonellosis *Agent:* *Salmonella* bacteria (more than 1700 types; Typhoid is one of these types).	May be in poultry, eggs, fish, raw meats, milk. Multiplies rapidly at room temperature.	*Symptoms:* Nausea, fever, headache, abdominal cramps (severe), diarrhea, sometimes vomiting. *Onset:* 12–48 hrs. after eating. Can be fatal in infants, elderly, infirm.	• Safe and sanitary food source. • Sanitary food-handling practices. • Thorough cooking of foods. • Proper and prompt refrigeration of foods. • Fish, shellfish from area waters contaminated with sewage to be avoided.
Botulism *Agent:* Botulinum toxin (produced by the *Clostridium botulinum* bacteria). *This illness is an intoxication and does not have intestinal symptoms.*	Bacteria widespread in environment; produces toxin only in *anaerobic* (oxygen-free) environment of little acidity. Types A, B, F may result from inadequate processing of low-acid canned foods, such as mushrooms, green beans, olives, beef. Type E in fish.	*Neurotoxic Symptoms:* Double vision, inability to swallow, hoarseness, speech difficulty, progressive paralysis of the respiratory system. *Call for medical help or transport to emergency room immediately! Botulism can be fatal.*	• Proper method for home canning low-acid foods. • Avoid commercially canned low-acid foods with leaky seals or with bent, bulging or broken cans. • Toxin is destroyed after a can is opened by *boiling contents hard for 10 minutes or more* (This is *not* recommended).

Hepatitis (Infectious; yellow jaundice) *Agent:* Hepatitis A virus (virus)	Infected human sewage; shellfish harvested in contaminated waters; food prepared or handled by infected personnel; contaminated water supplies.	*Symptoms:* Fatigue, malaise, nausea, vomiting, jaundice. *Onset:* 15–50 days. May cause liver damage; death.	• Safe and sanitary food source. • Approved source of shellfish. • Use of pure drinking water (intact supplies). • Proper and intact sewerage. • Adequate cooking of food. • Exclusion of infected food handlers.
Giardiasis *Agent: Giardia lamblia* (flagellate protozoa)	Untreated mountain streams and ponds (believed contaminated by animal reservoirs); human intestinal tracts (infected) contaminating food and water sources.	*Symptoms:* Sudden onset of watery diarrhea, flatulence, distention, nausea, anorexia, cramps, vomiting, foul sulfuric belching. *Onset:* 15 days.	• Avoiding unknown water supplies. • Avoiding raw fruits and vegetables in endemic areas. • Proper and intact sewerage. • Exclusion of infected food handlers. • Sanitary food handling.
Cholera *Agent: Vibrio cholera* (bacteria)	Bacteria in infected human feces; waters contaminated by human sewage; seafood harvested from waters contaminated with infected sewage.	*Symptoms:* May vary from mild, uncomplicated with diarrhea to intense diarrhea, dehydration, to fatal. *Onset:* 1–3 days.	• Proper sewage disposal. • Proper and intact sewerage. • Thorough cooking of seafood. • Sanitary handling of food. • Exclusion of infected food handlers.
Shigellosis (dysentery) *Agent: Shigella* (bacteria—many types)	Bacteria in infected human feces; waters contaminated by human sewage; food contaminated by infected food handler.	*Symptoms:* Abdominal cramps, fever, diarrhea, vomiting, may have blood and pus in feces. *Onset:* 1–7 days. Serious in infants, elderly, and debilitated patients.	• Proper sewage disposal. • Intact sewerage. • Sanitary food handling and food source. • Exclusion of infected food handlers.

Epidemiologists constantly are involved in studies of a variety of conditions in the area in which they work. By being constantly aware of the source of an agent, the transmission methods of that agent, and the routes that the agent may take, the epidemiologist has the key to open many doors of investigation. After studying the epidemic, the epidemiologist also has the power to implement control measures that are effective and protective of the population in the community. Through finding poor handling practices in a variety of areas—food preparation, water supply regulation, solid waste disposal, clinical or hospital practices—the epidemiologist may become a benefactor to these facilities by bringing forth his or her findings. By identifying suspect sources, the epidemiologist may put into motion the activity necessary to eliminate the agent and the source, thus bringing about the control of the present epidemic and perhaps preventing future epidemics. The finding of a small epidemic in a community can have far-reaching consequences if an item (e.g., a food product) is produced in a distant location or a foreign country. If the product manufacturer's market is large and reaches countries throughout the world, "small" epidemics can become numerous and spread further. An example of this type of far-reaching source of an agent was reported in 1965 by the Erie County Health Department after an outbreak of shigellosis occurred among hundreds of students at the State University of New York at Buffalo, who had consumed shrimp that had been imported from India (Elsea, Mosher, Lennon, Markellis, & Hoffman, 1971). Shortly following the outbreak, a small epidemic occurred in a small private school in Buffalo and the vehicle again was shrimp imported from the same source in India, but the agent was a type of salmonella. By curtailing any further selling of that particular product, other epidemics were prevented.

Because foodborne illnesses lend themselves to basic conditions for epidemiological study, Table 14.3 has been included for the purpose of instruction for beginning students of epidemiology. Table 14.3 consists of a listing of diseases and causative agents, sources, symptoms, and preventive methods of only a selected small number of these illnesses. Even though the selection is not extensive, the student should become aware of the variety of sources, agents, symptoms, and etiological agents. This will help to promote an understanding of the importance of knowing the symptoms and incubation times of each disease if one is to become a good epidemiologist investigating communicable diseases.

Epilog

Epidemiology and Strategies for Disease Prevention and Health Promotion

Epidemiology provides the intelligence on which public health campaigns can be based. Most of the early successes of public health relied on changing the environment—draining lowlands, installing sewers, establishing clean water supplies. Since Pasteur, vaccination has been responsible for some of our greatest successes, such as the eradication of smallpox and the drastic reductions in morbidity and mortality due to polio, diphtheria, whooping cough, and measles. Today, we are increasingly concerned with efforts to prevent disease and injury through behavior change, such as abstinence from smoking, moderation in use of alcohol, use of seat belts, and so forth. As each of these successes has reduced one threat to human life, we have gone on to challenge the next threat.

The First Epidemiologic Revolution[1]

In the 19th century, three-fifths of all deaths were due to infectious diseases. The leading causes of death in 1850 were tuberculosis, dysentery and diarrhea, cholera, malaria, typhoid fever, pneumonia,

[1]The discussion in this and the following section is based largely on the contributions of Dr. Milton Terris, distinguished epidemiologist and editor of the *Journal of Public Health Policy*.

diphtheria, scarlet fever, meningitis, whooping cough, measles, ery-sipelas, and smallpox. Parents could expect that half or more of their children would die of one of these or some other condition before reaching adulthood.

Sanitation measures aimed at providing pure water, milk, and food were responsible for the virtual disappearance of cholera, dysentery, and typhoid fever from the United States. These environmental mea-sures, in conjunction with well-baby clinics and health education for women, have largely eliminated infant diarrhea from the category of fatal conditions. Malaria was vulnerable to drainage of lowlands and economic change, which eliminated the many small millponds through the growth of central milling. Wartime efforts at insecticide spraying and medical treatment of infected persons, during World War II, helped finish the near elimination of malaria from the United States.

Social progress, including better housing and reduced overcrowding, has resulted in dramatic decreases in pneumonia, erysipelas, scarlet fever, and meningitis. In the past few decades, since antibiotics have become available, medical care has contributed marginally to the further reduction in death due to these causes. Smallpox, diphtheria, whooping cough, and measles all succumbed to mass immunization programs.

Tuberculosis declined as the labor unions grew and brought about a higher standard of living for American workers. Less crowding, housing with more sunlight and better ventilation, and better nutrition played the key roles in the decline of TB. Public health measures of case-finding and isolation also contributed to the decline in this killer. Finally, the development of effective drugs for the treatment of TB has, in the past few decades, given medicine a role in reducing this problem.

These major successes in reducing morbidity and mortality due to the infectious diseases represent what Milton Terris (1976; 1980) has called the first epidemiologic revolution. Success came largely through environmental measures aimed at controlling exposure to infectious agents and their vectors, and through vaccination against those agents. General improvements in the standard of living, resulting largely from unionization, also played an important role in the first epidemiologic revolution. Winslow (1923) points out that health education first emerged as a disease prevention strategy in the campaign against tuberculosis and was to play a critical role in every successful effort at improving the public's health thereafter. The role of medicine, until quite recently, was limited for the most part to reducing suffering— rarely having any capacity to either prevent or cure disease.

The Second Epidemiologic Revolution _____

Today, only about one in every 10 deaths is due to an infectious disease.[2] Cardiovascular diseases, including heart disease and stroke, accounted for 49 percent of all deaths in the United States in 1981. Cancer accounted for an additional 21 percent; accidents for 5 percent; and chronic obstructive lung disorders, such as asthma and emphysema, for nearly 3 percent. The remainder of the 12 leading causes of death were pneumonia and influenza, diabetes mellitus, chronic liver disease, suicide, homicide, birth defects, kidney disease, and septicemia (blood poisoning).

The challenge of the second epidemiologic revolution is to reduce  morbidity and mortality due to chronic and, for the most part, noninfectious diseases. Although some of the same strategies may be applicable, it seems clear that the second revolution will rely to a far greater degree on changing the behavior of individuals. And these changes, in many instances, will not be easy ones to accomplish. We are not simply encouraging hand washing or putting up screens; we are asking people to change very basic behaviors. In the words of Aaron Wildavsky (1976),

> We are not talking about peripheral or infrequent aspects of human behavior. We are talking about some of the most deeply rooted and often experienced aspects of human life—what one eats, how often and how much;... whether one smokes or drinks and how much; even the whole question of human personality.

Such a task is formidable. It also raises ethical concerns of grave importance about the right of society to encourage or even coerce certain lifestyle decisions and the right of an individual to persist in unhealthy behavior. No easy answers are likely to be found to either the ethical or the procedural questions that are being raised by the second epidemiologic revolution.

---

[2]However, it is possible that some diseases normally thought of as noninfectious may actually have infectious agents. Cancer, for instance, may have a viral agent. The same is true of diabetes mellitus. If these hypotheses are true, then infectious diseases account for about one-third of all deaths.

Strategies for Disease Prevention and Health Promotion

We may attempt to prevent disease or promote health through environmental change. This may involve draining a swamp, regulating materials used in construction or manufacturing, or organizing a union. On the other hand, our efforts may be aimed at changing the potential hosts of disease—either biologically or behaviorally. We may vaccinate or medicate potential hosts in order to increase their resistance to disease, or we may try to change their behavior in such a way as to reduce their exposure to causes of disease.

Whether our efforts are aimed at changing the environment or the potential hosts, we may attempt to do it for all or part of the community. A public health campaign may be community-wide or it may be focused on identified high-risk groups or environments. A third alternative is provided by milestone programs, in which, figuratively speaking, all the community marches past and all are affected when they pass by the milestone, for instance, requiring all 8th-grade students to have a health education class or vaccinating all 2-month-old children against measles.

Community-Wide Environmental Strategies

These approaches attempt to change the physical, biological, or social environment of the entire community. This may be attempted in order to reduce the exposure of potential hosts to agents or other harmful influences. Alternatively, it may be intended to increase the accessibility of resources that will strengthen the potential hosts' resistance to disease.

Swamp drainage, sewage disposal, and water purification systems are classic examples of this approach to reducing exposure to agents through the physical environment. Clean Indoor Air Acts, which forbid smoking in indoor public places, are variants on this classic approach. Crash barriers on public roadways are likewise examples of this approach. Spraying for mosquitoes to prevent the spread of malaria, yellow fever, or encephalitis is another example. Planting trees as a barrier to noise pollution is another instance in the realm of the biological environment. On the social front, efforts to eliminate racism, sexism, and ageism from our social institutions serve much the same purpose.

We may seek to alter the environment in order to make useful resources more accessible (e.g., by developing public recreation facilities to make opportunities for exercise, fresh air, and sunshine more available to the public). The biological environment may be enhanced by planting public gardens and planter boxes. The social environment may be enriched in many ways—the greatest of these being the institution of public schools.

The most common objection to these strategies is one of expense. It costs a lot to provide these services. Some people are certain to question whether some of these measures do not cost more than they are worth. Furthermore, although these measures are aimed at the whole community, not everyone makes any direct use of them. A public golf course, for instance, makes a healthful form of recreation available to the community as a whole. Nongolfers, however, may see it as a service to a minority of golfing doctors and businessmen that the general public is forced to pay for.

Community-Wide Host-Centered Strategies

Mass vaccination programs may be carried out in an attempt to immunize every potential host in the community. Mass media may be used to warn everyone of the dangers of smoking. We can put fluoride in everyone's drinking water in order to protect them against tooth decay. We can even raise the taxes on alcohol to discourage overconsumption.

In addition to the problems noted above for community-wide strategies, these strategies raise issues of freedom of choice. What right does society have, some ask, to coerce individual citizens not to smoke or drink, or to put fluoride in their water without their consent? Perhaps the more difficult issue is that even if we accept those interventions by society, where do we place the limits? If society can put fluoride in our water to prevent tooth decay, can it put contraceptive drugs in our water to control population? If it can discourage smoking with higher taxes, can it put a tax on obesity—so much tax per pound over the height/weight chart norms?

Environmental Milestone Strategies

Milestone strategies are a lower cost way of trying to reach an entire community. For instance, if we could ascertain that every car on the road was in safe operating condition, a great many accidents would be averted. But to go through a community and inspect every car in one day would be an enormous and expensive effort. Many states have instead required such an inspection annually before renewing license plates. Thus, in the course of a year every car is inspected.

In the truest sense of a milestone strategy, the milestone is reached only once in a lifetime. Such a true example would be the public health department approval of sewer systems. In this case, the milestone takes place during the construction of a home or other building. The sewer system plan, and often its actual installation, must be approved by the local public health authorities. In most cases, this will not be reinspected as long as it is not replaced, enlarged, or modified.

Milestone programs have the drawback that their effects may be considerably diminished as time passes after the milestone. A car that passed inspection last month may have a burnt-out turn signal light, a leaking brake line, or defective steering this month. The sewer plan that was approved and installed 5 years ago may be leaking raw sewage into the water table today.

Host-Centered Milestone Strategies

It is in programs aimed at potential hosts that milestone strategies are most often used. Immunization programs provide an excellent example. We recommend a schedule of vaccinations tied to the age of the child, for instance. In most states we back this up with a further milestone, requiring that all children must have certain vaccinations before entering school.

Health education programs have often been mandated to occur at certain grade levels, thus constituting an environmental approach. If all children must receive sex education in, perhaps, the 6th grade, and because we all pass through the 6th grade on our way to adulthood, then everyone will receive sex education before reaching adulthood. The problem with this approach is that the health practices people learn at one age do not necessarily continue to be practiced at a later age. The common assumption that the health behaviors learned early in life will stick with us throughout life has been repeatedly disproved.

Strategies for High-Risk Environments

We may focus our efforts on changing those environments where the risks are greatest. Community-organization strategies to empower the poor and powerless have often had powerful effects on reducing morbidity and mortality among the poor by improving their access to the resources needed for health maintenance and health restoration.

Other strategies may also be targeted on the high-risk environment. For instance, schistosomiasis is an important disease in many of the tropical regions of the world. The agent of the disease exits from its human host in urine or feces and infects freshwater snails; the agent exits the snails in a different form—a free-swimming larvae that can penetrate human skin and infect persons who are swimming or wading in the water. One way to control this problem is to build privies in high-risk areas so that people will be less likely to urinate or defecate in the water. Another way is to provide treated water for bathing, swimming, and so on in high-risk areas to keep people out of the contaminated streams. Yet another is to use pesticides to kill the snails in high-risk areas.

Strategies for High-Risk Groups

Utilizing the knowledge that we have gained from descriptive epidemiology and that we have confirmed in many instances through analytic epidemiology, we may identify groups of persons who are at high risk of disease or injury and offer special services to them. In recent years this strategy has become increasingly popular, both as a way of reducing costs and as a way of better justifying societal intervention into people's private lives. The children of alcoholics, for example, are at high risk of becoming alcoholics themselves, thus we might target them for alcohol education and psychological services aimed at preventing alcoholism. Prostitutes are at high risk of cervical cancer, so we might offer them frequent Pap smears for early detection of cervical cancer. Homosexual men are at high risk of AIDS, so we might focus educational and screening efforts on them.

The problem with this approach is that although we can clearly identify high-risk groups, it does not as readily apply to individuals. We can take a conservative approach, trying to identify only those who are very likely to develop the disease we are trying to prevent. In that case, we will leave out of our target group many if not most of those who will eventually develop the disease, thus limiting our impact. On the other hand, we can broadly include everyone whose risk is greater than the norm, in which case our target population becomes so large that this approach is not greatly less expensive than a community-wide strategy. For instance, Rogers (1968) studied the use of risk assessment in the early detection of children with handicapping conditions. He found that it was necessary to include 41 percent of the children in the high-risk group in order to include 65 percent of the children who later developed chronic handicaps. In a similar study of risk of mental retardation, Davie, Butler, and Goldstein (1972) found that it was necessary to include one-fourth of all newborns in the high-risk group in order for that group to contain 51 percent of the children who actually were identified as mentally retarded. Many more examples are possible.

A further problem with approaches that focus on high-risk groups or high-risk environments is stigmatization (Goffman, 1963). Being labeled as part of a "high-risk" group may have destructive social consequences for those so-labeled. Renewed discrimination against homosexuals because they are at high risk of AIDS is a current example. There is even the possibility, in some cases, of a "self-fulfilling prophecy," in which being labeled as "high risk" actually contributes to the development of the disease or condition. Services intended to prevent juvenile delinquency or drug abuse in high-risk youths may actually stigmatize those youths, cutting them off from socially desirable influences and increasing their exposure to harmful influences (Duncan, 1969; Foster, Dinitz, & Reckless, 1972).

The Need for Wellness Strategies _____

The progress that has been made in reducing morbidity and delaying mortality has allowed us to become aware that health is more than the mere absence of disease. This growing awareness was formalized in 1948, in the Constitution of the World Health Organization, which says:

> Health is a state of complete physical, mental and social well-being and not merely the absence of disease or infirmity.

There remains a tendency, however, to confuse health with its opposite, illness—as in such accepted usage as *health care* for the treatment of illness or *health center* for a place where the sick are brought together for treatment. Halbert L. Dunn (1961), therefore, coined the word *wellness* for a state of positive health and *high-level wellness* for the state of complete physical, mental, social, and spiritual well-being. A true epidemiology of health or wellness has not yet emerged but there have been efforts in that direction (Dunn, 1957; Terris, 1975)—such as the "Peckham Experiment" (Duncan, 1985)—

and the time seems ripe for the development of such a field in the near future.

Terris (1975) points out that the measurement of health status by epidemiologists has progressed

> from the most solidly established phenomenon, death, to include more severe illness, then mild illness, and finally health. The road traversed in this fashion has become progressively more difficult and uncertain. (p. 1038)

In proposing the next steps down that road, he suggests that an epidemiology of health might begin with studies of performance levels of population groups in relation to health factors; capacity for performance—physical and mental fitness; impediments to performance and the means to overcome them; and such subjective feelings as comfort, well-being, and vitality.

Dunn (1957) discusses nine "points of attack for raising the levels or wellness" in America. Briefly, these nine points are as follows:

1. Measures to improve wellness in family living and community life. A major element of this is the education of community caregivers, such as physicians, teachers, and clergymen, so as to recognize and encourage those factors that can be identified as promoting health, especially mental health.
2. Education, with more emphasis on teaching "wisdom" and good judgment than on teaching facts.
3. Human relations. Helping people to develop skills for cooperation and adjustment in facing life's problems.
4. Leadership. Focusing efforts at wellness promotion on those persons who influence the lives of many others.
5. Communication and access to information. "Perhaps there is nothing more important to a free society and well minds than open channels of communication and access to relevant information" (p. 231).
6. Creative expression. The importance placed by society on creative expression of all types should be enhanced.
7. Altruism. The value of altruism should be conscientiously promoted.
8. Maturity. This was a key concept to Dunn, which needed to be concretized in its broadest sense and promoted as the desired goal of all development.
9. Longevity. Extending the productive years of those who achieve maturity.

William Carlyon (1984), health educator for the American Medical Association, argues that health promotion has been hindered by a tendency to think in terms of a medical model and to confuse health promotion and wellness with disease prevention. He compares approaching wellness through risk reduction to "using a map of China to explore Africa" (p. 28).

> The core concept of wellness, according to our own rhetoric, is self-actualization and personal fulfillment. This in turn enables people to achieve a condition of wholeness, happiness, high-quality living—with dignity, purpose and meaning, alive clear to your fingertips, tingling with vitality. (p. 28)

Carlyon identifies the major barriers to wellness not as smoking or cholesterol, but as racism, sexism, and prejudice in all forms; bigotry, and intolerance; social Darwinism; the combat approach to human relations—competitiveness, anti-intellectualism, nationalism, and militarism. He warns that many wellness enthusiasts display just these attitudes, which they should be fighting against.

An epidemiology of wellness is emerging that can provide guidance to our efforts at health promotion but it will be concerned with far different health states than the mortality, morbidity, and disability measured by traditional disease-centered epidemiology. The epidemiology of wellness will be concerned with such health states and causal influences as love, creativity, humor, happiness, flexibility, self-esteem, and joy-of-living.

Recommended Readings _____

Carlyon, W. H. (1984). Disease prevention/health promotion—Bridging the gap to wellness. *Health Values, 8*(3), 27–30.

Duncan, D. F. (1985). The Peckham Experiment: A pioneering exploration of wellness. *Health Values, 9*(5), 40–43.

Duncan, D. F., & Gold, R. S. (Eds.). (1986). Special issue: Health promotion through the life cycle. *Health Values, 10*(3), entire issue.

Dunn, H. L. (1957). Points of attack for raising the levels of wellness. *Journal of the National Medical Association, 49,* 225–235.

Terris, M. (1975). Approaches to an epidemiology of health. *American Journal of Public Health, 65,* 1037–1045.

Terris, M. (1980). Epidemiology as a guide to health policy. *Annual Review of Public Health, 1,* 323–344.

References

Ardell, D. B. (1977). *High level wellness: An alternative to doctors, drugs, and diseases*. Emmaus, PA: Rodale Press.

Ardell, D. B. (1982). *Fourteen days to a wellness lifestyle*. Mill Valley, CA: Whatever Publishing.

Ast, D. B., & Schlesinger, E. R. (1956). The conclusion of a ten-year study of water fluoridation. *American Journal of Public Health, 46,* 265–271.

Baranowski, T. (1981). Toward the definition of concepts of health and disease, wellness and illness. *Health Values, 5*(6), 246–256.

Baric, L. (1969). Recognition of the "at-risk" role: A means to influence behavior. *International Journal of Health Education, 12,* 24–34.

Belloc, N. B., & Breslow, L. (1972). Relationships of physical health status and health practices. *Preventive Medicine, 1,* 409–421.

Berkman, L. F., & Breslow, L. (1983). *Health and ways of living*. New York: Oxford University Press.

Burke, J. (1978). *Connections*. Boston: Little, Brown & Company.

Campbell, D. T., & Stanley J. C. (1966). *Experimental and quasi-experimental designs for research*. Chicago: Rand McNally.

Carlyon, W. H. (1981). Myths, mindsets, and the medical model: Misunderstanding school health instruction. *Health Values, 5*(5), 207–210.

Carlyon, W. H. (1984). Disease prevention/health promotion—Bridging the gap to wellness. *Health Values, 8*(3), 27–30.

Cartwright, F. F. (1972). *Disease and history*. New York: New American Library.

Comstock, G. (1974). Commentary. In R. V. Kasius (Ed.), *The challenge of facts: Selected public health papers of Edgar Sydenstricker*. New York: Prodist.

Cook, T. D. & Campbell, D. T. (1979). *Quasi-experimentation*. Boston: Houghton Mifflin.

Cornfield, J. (1978). Randomization by group: A formal analysis. *American Journal of Epidemiology, 108,* 100–102.

Davie, R., Butler, N., & Goldstein, H. (1972). *From birth to seven*. London: Longman.

Derr, J. M. (1973). *Rural social problems, human services, and social policies* (Working Paper 10, Mental Health and Mental Retardation.) Denver: University of Denver, Center for Social Research and Development.

Dohrenwend, B. P., & Dohrenwend, B. S. (November, 1971). The prevalence of psychiatric disorders in urban vs. rural settings. *Proceedings of the Fifth World Congress of Psychiatry*, Mexico City, Mexico, November, 1971.

Dohrenwend, B. P., & Dohrenwend, B. S. (1982). Perspectives on the past and future of psychiatric epidemiology (The 1981 Rema Lapouse Lecture). *American Journal of Epidemiology, 72*, 1271–1279.

Donabedian, A. (1973). *Aspects of medical care administration*. Cambridge, MA: Harvard University Press.

Dubos, R. (1959). *Mirage of health*. Garden City, NY: Doubleday.

Dubos, R. (1965). *Man adapting*. New Haven: Yale University Press.

Duncan, D. F. (1969). Stigma and delinquency. *Cornell Journal of Social Relations, 4*(2), 41–48.

Duncan, D. F. (1985). The Peckham Experiment: A pioneering exploration of wellness. *Health Values, 9*(5), 40–43.

Duncan, D. F., & Gold, R. S. (1982). *Drugs and the whole person*. New York: Macmillan.

Duncan, D. F., & Gold, R. S. (1986). Health promotion: What is it? *Health Values, 10*(3), 47–48.

Dunham, H. W. (1965). *Community and schizophrenia: An epidemiological analysis*. Detroit: Wayne State University Press.

Dunham, H. W. (1970). Epidemiological research in schizophrenia. *Michigan Mental Health Research Bulletin, 4*(4), 7–16.

Dunham, H. W. (1986). Mental disorders in urban areas: A retrospective view. In M. M. Weissman, J. K. Myers, & C. E. Ross (Eds.), *Community surveys of psychiatric disorders*. New Brunswick, NJ: Rutgers University Press.

Dunn, H. L. (1957). Points of attack for raising the levels of wellness. *Journal of the National Medical Association, 49*, 225–235.

Dunn, H. L. (1959). What high-level wellness means. *Canadian Journal of Public Health, 50*, 447–457.

Dunn, H. L. (1961). *High level wellness*. Thorofare, NJ: Slack.

Eaton, W. W. (1985). *Epidemiologic field methods in psychiatry: The NIMH Epidemiologic Catchment Area Program*. Orlando, FL: Academic Press.

Edgerton, J. W., Bentz, W. K., & Hollister, W. G. (1970). Demographic factors and responses to stress among rural people. *American Journal of Public Health, 60*, 1065–1071.

Elsea, W. R., Mosher, W. E., Lennon, R. G., Markellis, V., & Hoffman, P. F. (1971). An epidemic of food-associated pharyngitis and diarrhea. *Archives of Environmental Health, 23*, 48–55.

Evans, A. S. (1978). Causation and disease: A chronological journey. *American Journal of Epidemiology, 108*, 249–258.

Faris, R. E. L., & Dunham, W. H. (1939). *Mental disorders in urban areas*. Chicago: University of Chicago Press.

Farquhar, J. W. (1978). The community-based model of life style intervention trials. *American Journal of Epidemiology, 108*, 103–111.

Farquhar, J. W., Fortmann, S. P., Maccoby, N., Haskell, W. L., Williams,

P. T., Flora, J. A., Taylor, C. B., Brown, B. W., Jr., Solomon, D. S., & Hulley, S. B. (1985). The Stanford Five-City Project: Design and methods. *American Journal of Epidemiology, 122,* 323–334.

Ferrara, C. P. (1980). *Vital and health statistics: Techniques of community health analysis.* Atlanta: Centers for Disease Control.

Foster, J. D., Dinitz, S., & Reckless, W. C. (1972). Perceptions of stigma following public intervention for delinquent behavior. *Social Problems, 20,* 20–22.

Fox, J. P., Hall, C. E., & Elveback, L. R. (1970). *Epidemiology: Man and disease.* New York: Macmillan.

Friedman, G. D. (1980). *Primer of epidemiology.* New York: McGraw-Hill.

Friedman, M. (1984). The history of an idea. In M. Friedman, & D. Ulmer, *Treating Type A behavior and your heart.* New York: Alfred A. Knopf.

Furcolow, M. L. (1962). Serological evidence of histoplasmosis in sanitoriums in the U.S. *Journal of the American Medical Association, 180,* 109–114.

Gibson, R., Schuman, L., & Bjelke, E. (1985). *A prospective study of coffee consumption and mortality from cancer.* Paper presented at the Eighteenth Annual Meeting of the Society for Epidemiologic Research, Chapel Hill, NC.

Goffman, E. (1963). *Stigma: Notes on the management of spoiled identity.* Englewood Cliffs, NJ: Prentice-Hall.

Goldberger, J. (1914). The etiology of pellagra. *Public Health Reports, 29,* 1683–1686.

Gordon, T., & Kannel, W. B. (1984). Drinking and mortality: The Framingham Study. *American Journal of Epidemiology, 120,* 97–107.

Haberberger, R. L., Jr., Duncan, D. F., Frisch, L. E., & Narve, M. D. (1985). Epidemiological and clinical correlates of endocervical chlamydial infections in female college students presenting for routine pap examination. *Journal of American College Health, 33,* 262–263.

Hanlon, J. J., & Pickett, G. E. (1979). *Public health: Administration and practice.* St. Louis, MO: C. V. Mosby.

Hawkins, W. E., & Duncan, D. F. (1985a). Perpetrator and family characteristics related to child abuse and neglect: Comparison of substantiated and unsubstantiated reports. *Psychological Reports, 56,* 407–410.

Hawkins, W. E., & Duncan, D. F. (1985b). Children's illnesses as risk factors for child abuse. *Psychological Reports, 56,* 638.

Healthy People: The Surgeon General's Report on Health Promotion and Disease Prevention. (1979). Washington, DC: U.S. Government Printing Office.

Holmes. T. H., & Rahe, R. (1967). The Social Readjustment Rating Scale. *Journal of Psychosomatic Research, 11,* 213–218.

Hull, D. (1977). Life circumstances and physical illness. *Journal of Psychosomatic Research, 21,* 115–139.

Hutt, M. S. R., & Burkitt, D. P. (1986). *The geography of non-infectious disease.* Oxford: Oxford University Press.

Jenkins, C. D. (1976). Recent evidence supporting psychologic and social risk factors for coronary disease. *New England Journal of Medicine, 294,* 987–994 & 1033–1038.

Justice, B. (1987). *Who gets sick: Thinking and health.* Houston: Peak Press.

Justice, B., & Duncan, D. F. (1975). Physical abuse of children as a public health problem. *Public Health Review, 4,* 183–200.

Justice, B., & Duncan, D. F. (1976). Life crisis as a precursor to child abuse. *Public Health Reports, 91,* 110–115.

Justice, B., & Duncan, D. F. (1977). Child abuse in terms of a public health model. *Mental Health and Society, 4,* 110–114.

Justice, B., & Justice, R. (1976). *The abusing family.* New York: Human Sciences Press.

Kahn, H. A. (1983). *An Introduction to epidemiologic methods.* New York: Oxford University Press.

Kasl, S. V., & Cobb, S. (1966a). Health behavior, illness behavior, and sick role behavior: I. Health and illness behavior. *Archives of Environmental Health, 12,* 246–266.

Kasl, S. V., & Cobb, S. (1966b). Health behavior, illness behavior, and sick-role behavior: II. Sick-role behavior. *Archives of Environmental Health, 12,* 531–541.

Keller, P. A., Feil, R. N., Zimbelman, K. K., & Wenger, N. (1979). *A comparison of rural and urban suicide rates in the Northeastern United States.* (Mansfield Rural Community Psychology Paper 79-01.) Mansfield: Mansfield State College.

Koch, R. Ueber bakteriologische forschung. *Proceedings of the Tenth International Medical Conference.* Berlin.

Kolbe, L. J. (1983). Improving the health status of children: An epidemiological approach to establishing priorities for behavioral research. In *Proceedings of the National Conference on Research and Development in Health Education with Special Reference to Youth.* Southampton, England: Southampton University Press.

Levine, S., & Lilienfeld, A. M. (1987). *Epidemiology and health policy.* New York: Tavistock Publications.

Lilienfeld, A. M. (1960). The distribution of disease in the population. *Journal of Chronic Diseases, 11,* 471–483.

Lilienfeld, A. M. (1977). Epidemiology of infectious and non-infectious disease: Some comparisons. The First Wade Hampton Frost Lecture. *American Journal of Epidemiology, 97,* 135–147.

Lilienfeld, D. E. (1978). Definitions of epidemiology. *American Journal of Epidemiology, 107,* 87–90.

Lind, J. (1753). *A treatise of the scurvy.* Edinburgh: Sands, Murray and Cochran.

Maccoby, N., Farquhar, J. W., Wood, P. D., & Alexander, J. (1977). Reducing the risk of cardiovascular disease: Effects of a community-based campaign on knowledge and behavior. *Journal of Community Health, 3,* 100–114.

MacMahon, B., Pugh, T. F., & Ipsen, J. (1960). *Epidemiologic methods.* Boston: Little, Brown & Company.

Maslow, A. H. (1956). Self-actualizing people: A study of psychological health. In C. E. Moustakas (ed.), *The self: Explorations in personal growth.* New York: Harper and Row.

Maslow, A. H. (1970). *Motivation and personality* (2nd ed.). New York: Harper and Row.

Mason, T. J., Fraumeni, J. F., Jr., Hoover, R., & Blot, W. J. (1981). *An atlas of mortality from selected causes.* (DHEW Publication No. NIH 81-2397.) Washington, DC: U.S. Government Printing Office.

Mason, T. J., McKay, F. W., Hoover, R., Blot, W. J., & Fraumeni, J. F., Jr. (1975). *Atlas of cancer mortality for U.S. counties: 1950–1969.* (DHEW Publication No. NIH 75-780.) Washington, DC: U.S. Government Printing Office.

Mason, T. J., McKay, F. W., Hoover, R., Blot, W. J., & Fraumeni, J. F., Jr. (1976). *Atlas of cancer mortality among U.S. nonwhites: 1950–1969.* (DHEW Publication No. NIH 76-1204.) Washington, DC: Government Printing Office.

Menzel, H. (1950). Comment on Robinson's ecological correlations and the behavior of individuals. *American Sociological Review, 15,* 674.

Miettinen, O. S. (1985). *Theoretical epidemiology: Principles of occurrence research in medicine.* New York: John Wiley & Sons.

Morris, J. N. (1975). *Uses of epidemiology* (3rd ed.). New York: Churchill Livingstone.

MRFIT Research Group. (1982). Multiple risk factor intervention trial: Risk factor changes and mortality results. *Journal of the American Medical Association, 244,* 1465–1477.

Mullen, K. D. (1982). *Wellness constructs: A decision theoretic study.* Unpublished dissertation, Southern Illinois University, Carbondale.

Mullner, R. M., Byre, C. S., & Killingsworth, C. L. (1983). An inventory of U.S. health care data bases. *Review of Public Data Use, 11,* 85–192.

Myerson, A. (1940). Review of mental disorders in urban areas. *American Journal of Psychiatry, 16,* 995–997.

National Center for Health Statistics. (1985). *Health, United States, 1985* (DHHS Publication No. PHS 86-1232). Washington, DC: U.S. Government Printing Office.

Parsons, T. (1951). Social structure and dynamic process: The case of modern medical practice. In T. Parsons (Ed.), *The social system.* New York: Free Press.

Pearce, N. D. (1985). Health information resources: United States—health and social factors. In W. W. Holland, R. Detels, & G. Knox (Eds.), *Oxford Textbook of Public Health, Volume 3.* Oxford: Oxford University Press.

Peterson, D. R. & Thomas, D. B. (1978). *Fundamentals of epidemiology.* Lexington, MA: Lexington Books.

Regier, D. A. (1982). Progress in mental health epidemiology research. In M. O. Wagenfeld, P. V. Lemkau, & B. Justice (Eds.), *Perspective on public mental health.* Los Angeles: Sage.

Rhoads, G. G. (1984). The role of the case-control study in evaluating health interventions: Vitamin supplementation and neural tube defects. *American Journal of Epidemiology, 120,* 803–808.

Rice, D. (1985). Addendum—Health information systems: An overview. In W. W. Holland, R. Detels, & G. Knox (Eds.), *Oxford Textbook of Public Health, Volume 3.* Oxford: Oxford University Press.

Rice, J. E., & Duncan, D. F. (1985). Health practices and mental health: An exploratory study. *Psychological Reports, 57,* 1110.

Rindge, M. E. (1962). Infectious hepatitis: Report of an outbreak in a small Connecticut school due to water-borne transmission. *Journal of the American Medical Association, 180,* 33–37.

Robins, L. N. (1978). Psychiatric epidemiology. *Archives of General Psychiatry, 35,* 697–702.

Robins, L. N. (November, 1979). *Psychiatric diagnosis in the community: How and why?* Rema Lapouse Award Lecture presented to the 107th Annual Meeting of the American Public Health Association, New York, NY.

Robinson, W. S. (1950). Ecological correlation and the behavior of individuals. *American Sociological Review, 15,* 351–357.

Rogers, C. (1961). *On becoming a person.* Boston: Houghton Mifflin.

Rogers, M. (1968). Risk registers and the early detection of handicaps. *Developmental Medicine and Child Neurology, 10,* 651–661.

Ryan, R. S., & Travis, J. W. (1981) *The wellness workbook* (2nd ed.). Berkeley, CA: Ten Speed Press.

Scheuch, E. K. (1966). Cross-national comparisons using aggregate data: Some substantive and methodological problems. In R. L. Merritt & S. Rokkan (Eds.), *Comparing Nations.* New Haven: Yale University Press.

Schwab, J. J., Warheit, G., & Holzer, C. (1974). Mental health: Rural-urban comparisons. *Mental Health and Society, 1,* 254–274.

Seltser, R., & Sartwell, P. E. (1965). The influence of occupational exposure to radiation on the mortality of American radiologists and other medical specialists. *American Journal of Epidemiology, 81,* 2–22.

Sherwin, R. (1978). Controlled trials of the diet-heart hypothesis: Some comments on the experimental unit. *American Journal of Epidemiology, 108,* 92–99.

Siscovick, D. S., Weiss, N. S. & Fox, N. (1986). Moderate alcohol consumption and primary cardiac arrest. *American Journal of Epidemiology, 123,* 499–503.

Sizemore, J., & Duncan, D. F. (1986). Psychosocial epidemiology of rheumatoid arthritis in a rural population. *Psychological Reports, 59,* 866.

Smith, T. (1934). *Parasitism and disease.* Princeton, NJ: Princeton University Press.

Snow, J. (1855). On the mode of communication of cholera (2nd ed.). London: Churchill. (Reproduced in *Snow on Cholera,* New York: The Commonwealth Fund, 1936.)

Snow, J. (1936). *Snow on Cholera.* New York: The Commonwealth Fund.

Srole, L. (1972). Urbanization and mental health: Some reformulations. *American Scientist, 60,* 576–583.

Srole, L. (1978). The city versus town and country: New evidence on an ancient bias. In L. Srole & A. K. Fischer (Eds.), *Mental health in the metropolis: The midtown Manhattan study* (Book 2, rev. ed.). New York: Harper and Row.

Srole, L., & Fischer, A. K. (1980). Debate on psychiatric epidemiology. *Archives of General Psychiatry, 37,* 1421–1426.

Stallones, R. A. (1966). Prospective epidemiologic studies of cerebrovascular disease. *Public Health Monograph No. 76.* Washington, DC: U.S. Government Printing Office.

Stallones, R. A. (1980). To advance epidemiology. *Annual Review of Public Health, 1,* 69–82.

Stallones, R. A. (1983). Mortality and the multiple risk factor intervention trial. *American Journal of Epidemiology, 117,* 647–650.

Susser, M. (1973). *Causal thinking in the health sciences: Concepts and strategies of epidemiology.* New York: Oxford University Press.

Terris, M. (1962). The scope and methods of epidemiology. *American Journal of Public Health, 52,* 1371–1376.

Terris, M. (1975). Approaches to an epidemiology of health. *American Journal of Public Health, 65,* 1037–1045.

Terris, M. (1976). The epidemiologic revolution, national health insurance and the role of health departments. *American Journal of Public Health, 66,* 1155–1164.

Terris, M. (1980). Epidemiology as a guide to health policy *Annual Review of Public Health, 1,* 323–344.

Travis, J. (1981). *Wellness workbook.* Berkeley, CA: Ten Speed Press.

Wildavsky, A. (1976). *Can health be planned?* The Davis Lecture. Chicago: Center for Health Administration Studies, University of Chicago.

Winslow, C. -E. A. (1923). *The evolution and significance of the modern public health campaign.* New Haven: Yale University Press.

Winslow, C. -E. A. (1984). The evolution and significance of the modern public health campaign. South Burlington, VT: *Journal of Public Health Policy.*

Zinsser, H. (1942). *Rats, lice, and history,* (4th ed.). London: George Routledge.

Zunzunegui, M. V., King, M. -C., Coria, C. F. & Chalet, J. (1986). Male influences on cervical cancer risk. *American Journal of Epidemiology, 123,* 302–307.

Glossary

Adjusted Rate. Any rate that has been mathematically transformed to eliminate the influence of one or more variables—most often age.

Agent. An organism, substance, or force whose excess presence or relative absence is necessary for a particular disease to occur.

Bed-Disability Days. Days on which one stays in bed due to illness.

Confounding. A situation in which the effects of two variables are not separable.

Crude Rate. Summary rate based on the actual number of events in a total population over a given period of time.

Disability. Any restriction or lack of ability to perform an activity in the manner or within the range considered normal for human beings.

Epidemiology. The science that studies the distribution and determinants of varying rates of diseases, injuries, and health states in human populations.

Fomite. Personal article—such as handkerchiefs, toothbrushes, drinking glasses—that, if shared, may carry agents from host to host due to the relatively intimate contact with it.

General Fertility Rate (GFR). The ratio of live births to the number of women of childbearing age (usually assumed to be 15–44 years of age). The rate at which women in the population are having babies.

Gross Reproduction Rate (GRR). The ratio of female live births to the number of women of childbearing age (15–44).

Handicap. A disadvantage for any individual, resulting from a disability, that limits or prevents the fulfillment of a role that would be considered normal for that individual (given the individual's age, sex, social status, and so on).

Health. A state of complete physical, mental, and social well-being, and *not* the mere absence of disease or infirmity.

Health Maintenance. Measures targeted at disease-free individuals with the aim of preventing the occurrence of disease; primary prevention.

Health Promotion. Measures targeted at disease-free individuals with the aim of enhancing their level of wellness.

Health Restoration. Measures targeted at diseased individuals with the aim of restoring them to good health.

Host. The person (or other organism) in which the disease process takes place.

Impairment. Any loss or abnormality of psychological, physiological, or anatomical nature.

Incidence. The rate of new cases. The rate at which a disease spreads.

Infectivity. The ability of an agent to invade and reproduce itself in an exposed host.

Lifetime Prevalence. The proportion of persons within a population who have ever suffered from the disease or condition of interest.

Morbidity. Statistics on cases of disease.

Mortality. Statistics on deaths.

Natality. Statistics on births.

Neonatal Period. The first 28 days of life.

Net Reproduction Rate (NRR). The ratio of female live births minus female infant mortality in relation to the number of women of childbearing age (15–44). A more accurate approximation than gross reproduction rate of the rate at which women are giving birth to their own replacements in the population.

Odds Ratio. An approximation of relative risk calculatable from case-control studies; also known as relative odds.

Pathogenicity. The ability of an agent to produce disease in an infected host.

Perinatal Period. The period around the birth of a child. Perinatal period I extends from 28 weeks after conception until 1 week after birth. Perinatal period II extends from 20 weeks after conception until 4 weeks after birth.

Period Prevalence. The rate of current cases during some defined period of time.

Point Prevalence. The rate of current cases on one particular day.

Postneonatal Period. The period after the first 28 days of life but before the infant is 1 year old.

Prevalence. The rate of current cases (whether new or not) in a population. Rate expressing the proportion of the population at risk who suffered a given disease during a given time.

Primary Prevention. Keeping disease from occurring in the first place; aims to lower incidence by keeping new cases from occurring.

Rate. An expression of the proportion of some population who experienced a specified event.

Ratio. An expression of the relationship between two quantities.

Relative Odds. An approximation of relative risk calculatable from case-control studies; also known as odds ratio.

Relative Risk. The ratio of the risk of disease (incidence rate) among those exposed to some risk factor to the risk among the unexposed; also known as risk ratio.

Restricted-Activity Days. Days on which one reduces the range of activities due to illness.

Secondary Prevention. Early detection and treatment of disease; aims to lower prevalence by reducing the average duration of disease.

Secular Trend. A pattern of continuing increase or decrease over a period of 10 years or more.

Significance. The degree to which one can be certain that two measures are truly different and not the result of random errors in measurement. A significant difference is presumed to be a real difference; a nonsignificant difference is presumed to be a measurement or sampling error and thus no real difference exists.

Tertiary Prevention. The prevention of death or other long-term after-effects of illness.

Total Fertility Rate (TFR). The sum of annual age-specific birth rates for women aged 10–49. A more accurate estimate than general fertility rate of the rate at which women are having babies.

Vector. Originally, a blood-sucking insect that carries a disease agent from host to host. Now, generally used for any animal that thus carries disease and sometimes for nonliving vehicles of infection as well.

Vehicle. Any nonliving object or substance that carries an agent from host to host, such as fomites, water, or food.

Virulence. The ability of an agent to produce severe disease in a diseased host.

Vital Statistics. Records of the numbers of births, marriages, divorces, and deaths; sometimes used to mean all health-related statistics.

Index